Thoracic Radiology

Iacopo Carbone • Michele Anzidei
Editors

Thoracic Radiology

A Guide for Beginners

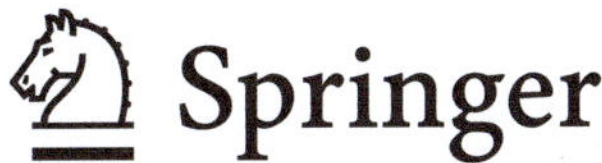

Editors
Iacopo Carbone
Department of Radiological, Oncological and Pathological Sciences
Sapienza, University of Rome
Rome
Italy

Head of Academic Diagnostic Imaging Division
I.C.O.T. Hospital
Latina
Italy

Michele Anzidei
Department of Radiological, Oncological and Pathological Sciences
Sapienza, University of Rome
Rome
Italy

ISBN 978-3-030-35764-1 ISBN 978-3-030-35765-8 (eBook)
https://doi.org/10.1007/978-3-030-35765-8

This Springer imprint is published by the registered company Springer Nature Switzerland AG
The registered company address is: Gewerbestrasse 11, 6330 Cham, Switzerland

To Livia, Anna, Caterina, Raffaello and Lucia: the bright stars of my own private sky.

Iacopo Carbone

Acknowledgement

The Editors and Authors would like to acknowledge the invaluable support given by their colleagues Christina Marrocchio, Susan Dababou, and Hans-Peter Erasmus who, besides contributing as chapter authors, worked at the revision and completion of the English manuscripts towards publication of this guide.

Without their engagement, the book would not have been possible.

Contents

Anatomy of the Thorax

1

Isabella Ceravolo, Michele Anzidei, and Susan Dababou

Trachea and Main Bronchi (Fig. 1.1)

The trachea has a cylindrical shape flattened posteriorly and is composed of 15–20 cartilaginous rings joined together by annular ligaments.

The trachea originates at the level of the C6–C7 vertebrae about 4 cm below the hyoid bone, extends for about 10–12 cm and branches into right and left main

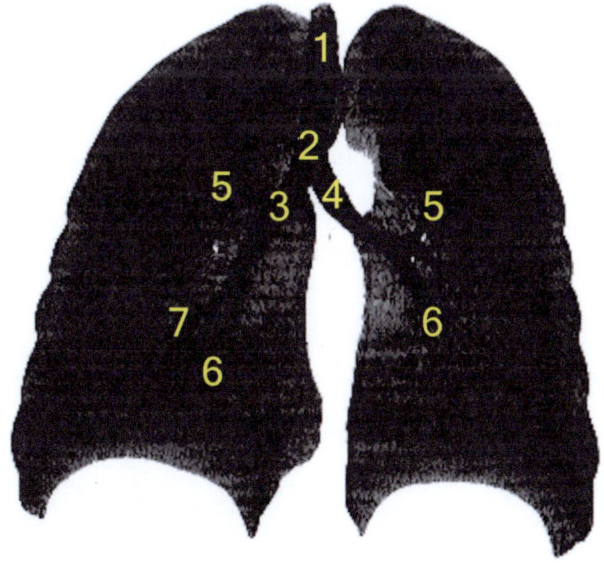

Fig. 1.1 (1) Trachea, (2) Carina of trachea, (3) Right bronchus, (4) Left bronchus, (5) Superior lobar bronchus, (6) Inferior lobar bronchus, (7) Middle lobar bronchus

I. Ceravolo · M. Anzidei · S. Dababou (✉)
Department of Radiological, Oncological and Pathological Sciences, Sapienza University of Rome, Rome, Italy

I. Carbone, M. Anzidei (eds.), *Thoracic Radiology*,
https://doi.org/10.1007/978-3-030-35765-8_1

bronchi at the level of T3–T4. This reference point at the base of the trachea is known as the carina.

Fissures and Lung Lobes

Lung fissures divide the lung parenchyma in anatomically and functionally independent lobes. The left lung is composed of two lobes (upper and lower) demarcated by the oblique fissure. The right lung has three lobes (upper, middle, and lower) separated by two fissures: the minor fissure (or horizontal fissure), which passes horizontally between the upper and middle lobes, and the major fissure (or oblique fissure), which separates the upper and middle lobes from the lower lobe (Figs. 1.2, 1.3, and 1.4).

Bronchopulmonary Segments (Fig. 1.5)

Bronchopulmonary segments are anatomically and functionally independent units within the lobes with an own ventilation (segment of the bronchus), vascular supply (branches of the pulmonary artery) and venous drainage. The anatomy of the bronchi and segments is illustrated in Figs. 1.6 and 1.7.

Mediastinal Compartments (Fig. 1.8)

The mediastinum is located in the median portion of the thorax and is bounded by the sternum and vertebral column anteroposteriorly, the mediastinal portion of the parietal pleura of both lungs laterally, the diaphragm inferiorly and by a horizontal plane passing through the first thoracic vertebra and the superior margin of the first rib superiorly. The mediastinum can be divided into four compartments:

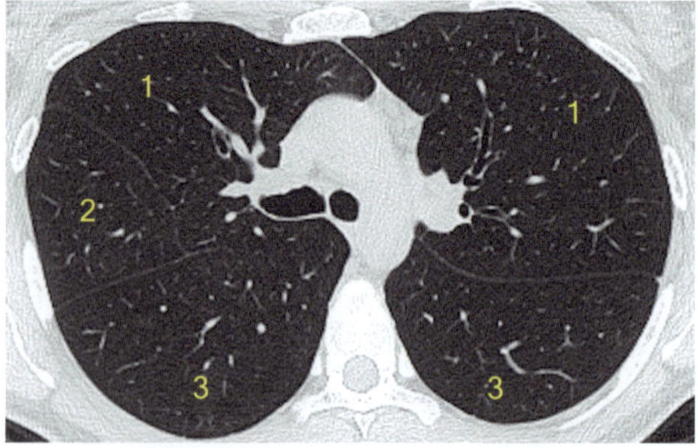

Fig. 1.2 (1) Upper lobe, (2) Middle lobe, (3) Lower lobe

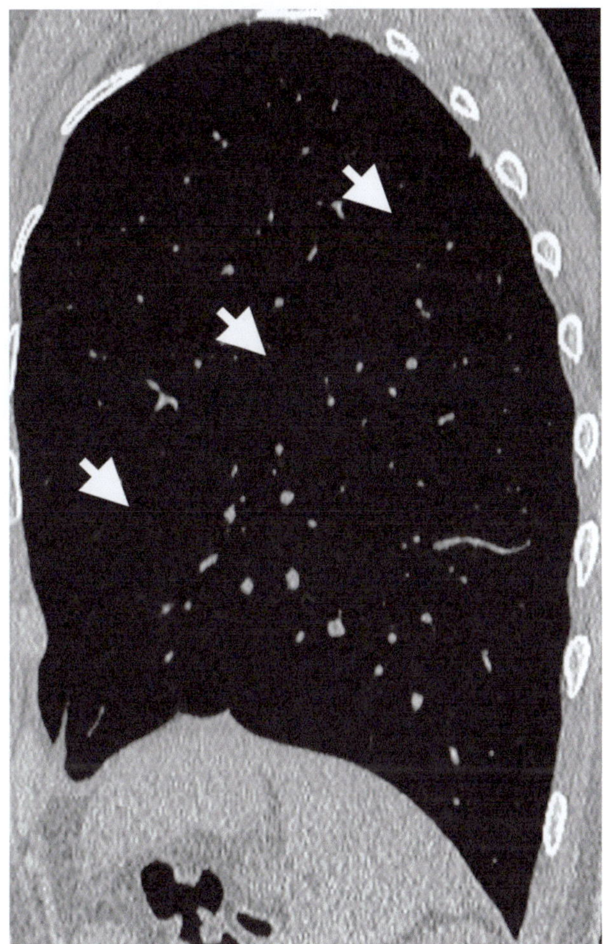

Fig. 1.3 CT scan, left lung lobe—The major fissure, or oblique fissure, (*white arrows*) originates in the superior portion of the hilum, runs upwards and backwards, passes the posterior margin, crosses the lateral surface, and descends obliquely up to the base. Then, it crosses the base and continues on the medial surface to end in the inferior part of the hilum

- The **anterior mediastinum** (prevascular space) includes the thymus, internal mammary vessels, pericardium, sternopericardial ligaments, loose connective tissue, and lymph nodes.
- The **superior mediastinum** contains the aortic arch, brachiocephalic trunk, left common carotid artery, left subclavian artery, the upper parts of the superior vena cava, thoracic duct, esophagus and trachea, lymph nodes, and adipose tissue.
- In the **middle mediastinum** (vascular space) we can find the heart, pericardium, ascending aorta, pulmonary arteries and veins, superior and inferior vena cava, the phrenic, vagus and recurrent laryngeal nerves, the carina, main bronchi, and lymph nodes.
- The **posterior mediastinum** contains the descending aorta, esophagus, thoracic duct, azygos and hemiazygos veins, nervous structures, and lymph nodes.

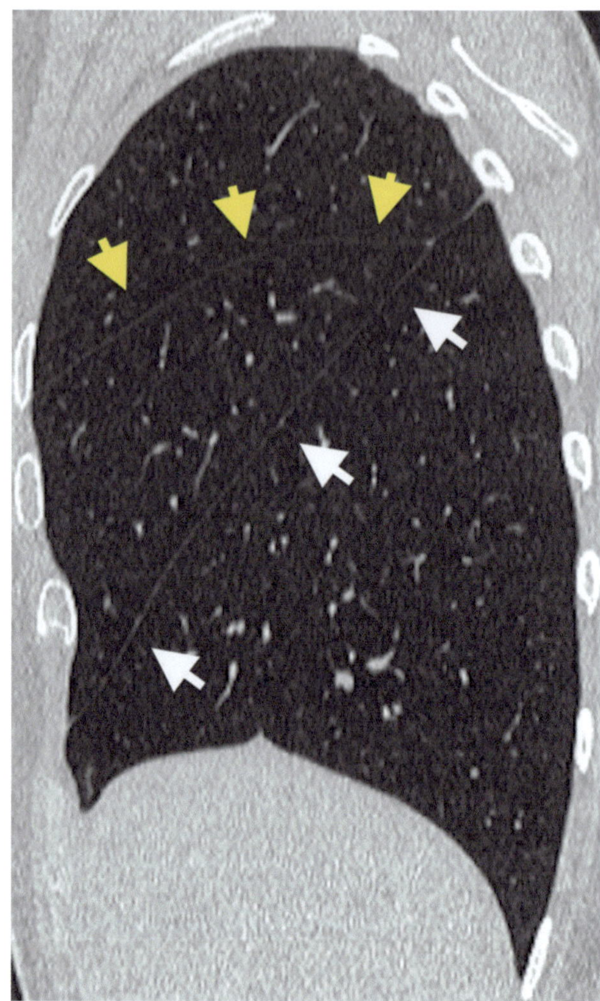

Fig. 1.4 CT scan, right lung lobe—The oblique fissure (*white arrows*) separates the upper and middle lobes form the lower lobe. The minor fissure, or horizontal fissure (*yellow arrow*), separates the right upper lobe from the middle lobe. The horizontal fissure separates from the oblique fissure at the level of the fourth rib, crosses horizontally the lateral surface of the lung, passes the anterior margin, and runs obliquely upwards ending at the hilum

Lymph Node Stations

Recognizing lymph node stations is crucial to stage cancers and decide the correct therapeutic approach. In 2014, the International Association for the Study of Lung Cancer (IASLC) proposed the following map for assessing lymph node stations (Figs. 1.9 and 1.10):

Supraclavicular Zone

Station 1: Low cervical, supraclavicular, and sternal notch lymph nodes—Station 1 is limited by the inferior margin of the cricoid cartilage superiorly and by

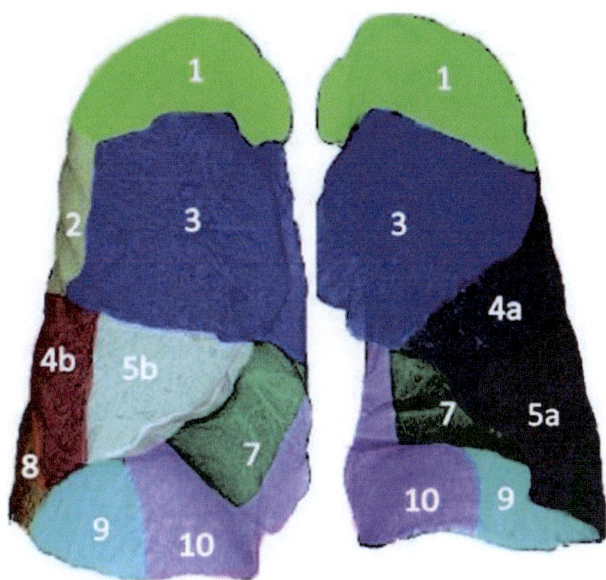

Fig. 1.5 Right Lung. Upper lobe: (1) Apical segment, (2) Posterior segment, (3) Anterior segment. Middle lobe: (4b) Lateral segment, (5b) Medial segment. Lower lobe: (8) Anterior basal segment, (9) Lateral basal segment, (7) Medial basal segment, (10) Posterior basal segment. Left Lung. Upper lobe: (1) Apicoposterior segment, (3) Anterior segment, (4a) Superior lingular segment, (5a) Inferior lingular segment. Lower lobe: (7) Anteromedial basal segment, (9) Lateral basal segment, (10) Posterior basal segment

the clavicles and the superior margin of the manubrium inferiorly. The median axis of the trachea separates the right and left lymph node stations.

Upper Zone

Station 2R: Right upper paratracheal lymph nodes—The superior border of this region is the apex of the right lung laterally and the superior border of the manubrium medially. The inferior border corresponds to the plane passing through the intersection between the caudal margin of the brachiocephalic vein and the median axis of the trachea.

Station 2L: Left upper paratracheal lymph nodes—The superior border is the apex of the left lung laterally and the superior border of the manubrium medially. The inferior border is at the level of the superior margin of the aortic arch.

Station 3A: Prevascular lymph nodes—The superior border of the prevascular zone is the thoracic apex, whereas the inferior border is at the level of the carina. Anteriorly, it is delimited by the posterior wall of the sternum; posteriorly, it is limited by the anterior border of the superior vena cava on the right and by the carotid artery on the left.

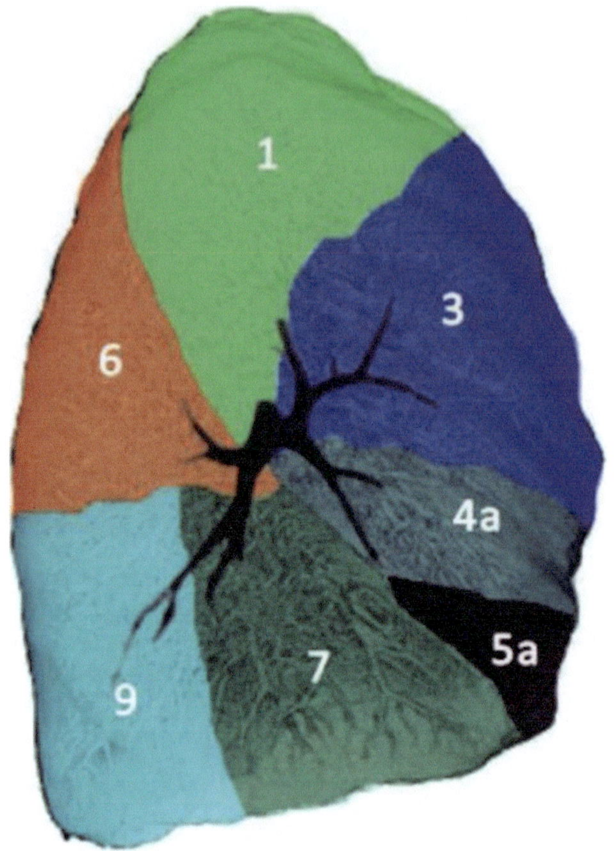

Fig. 1.6 Left Lung. Upper lobe: (1) Apicoposterior, (3) Anterior, (4a) Superior lingular, (5a) Inferior lingular. Lower lobe: (6) Superior, (7) Anteromedial basal, (9) Lateral basal

Station 3P: Retrotracheal lymph nodes—These lymph nodes are located in the retrotracheal space. The superior boundary of this region is the thoracic apex, the inferior one is at the level of the carina.

Station 4R: Right lower paratracheal lymph nodes—This region is bounded by the intersection between the margin of the brachiocephalic vein and the trachea superiorly and by the inferior margin of the azygos vein inferiorly.

Station 4L: Left lower paratracheal lymph nodes—The upper edge is the superior margin of the aortic arch. The lower one is the superior margin of the left pulmonary artery.

Aortopulmonary Zone

Station 5: Subaortic lymph nodes—The upper border of the aortopulmonary window is the inferior margin of the aortic arch, and the lower border is the superior margin of the left pulmonary artery.

Station 6: Para-aortic lymph nodes—These nodes run anterolaterally to the ascending aorta and the aortic arch.

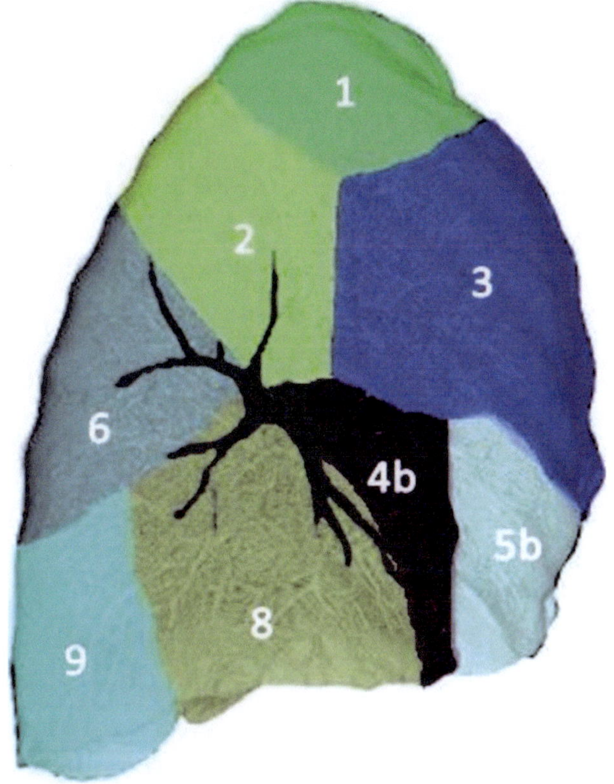

Fig. 1.7 Right Lung. Upper lobe: (1) Apical, (3) Anterior, (2) Posterior. Middle lobe: (4b) Lateral, (5b) Medial. Lower lobe: (6) Superior, (8) Anterior basal, (9) Lateral basal

Subcarinal Zone

Station 7: Subcarinal lymph nodes—The upper border is the carina and the inferior margin of the trachea. The edge of the lower bronchus on the left and of the intermediate bronchus on the right constitute the lower border.

Lower Zone

Station 8: Paraesophageal lymph nodes—They lie adjacent to the esophagus, extending from the inferior margin of the left lower and the right intermediate bronchus to the diaphragm.

Station 9: Pulmonary ligament lymph nodes—They are located along the pulmonary ligament, from the inferior pulmonary vein to the diaphragm.

Hilar and Interlobar Zone

Station 10: Hilar lymph nodes—They descend adjacent to the main bronchi and the hilar vessels. Superiorly, they extend to the lower margin of the azygos vein on

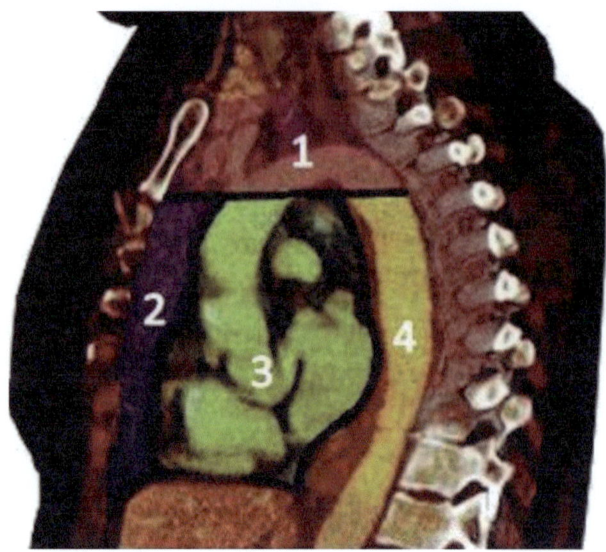

Fig. 1.8 (1) Superior mediastinum, (2) Anterior mediastinum, (3) Middle mediastinum, (4) Posterior mediastinum

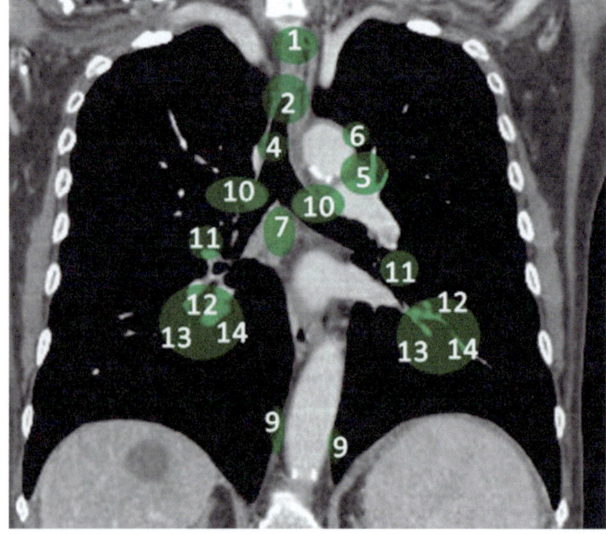

Fig. 1.9 (1) Sternal/supraclavicular, (2) Upper paratracheal, (4) Lower paratracheal, (5) Subaortic, (6) Para-aortic, (7) Subcarinal, (9) Pulmonary ligament, (10) Hilar, (11) Interlobar, (12) Lobar, (13) Segmental, (14) Subsegmental

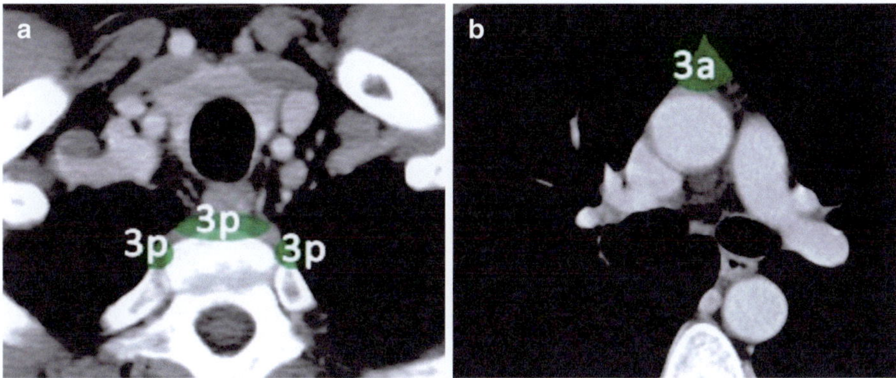

Fig. 1.10 Chest CT images identifying on the left (**a**) the Prevascular lymph nodes (3a), and on the right (**b**) the Retrotracheal lymph nodes (3p)

the right and to the upper margin of the pulmonary artery on the left. Inferiorly, they reach the interlobar regions.

Station 11: Interlobar lymph nodes—They are distributed along the origin of lobar bronchi. On the right, a further subdivision is made for lymph nodes located between upper and middle lobe, and middle and lower lobe.

Peripheral Zone

Stations 12, 13, 14: Lobar, segmental, and subsegmental lymph nodes—They follow the lobar, segmental, and subsegmental bronchi bilaterally.

Visualizing the Anatomy

The following pages show a series of axial chest CT scans (Figs. 1.11, 1.12, 1.13, 1.14, 1.15, 1.16, 1.17). Figure 1.11 identifies the main vascular structures. Figures 1.12 to 1.16 are couples of sequential axial chest CT scans, these consist of one lung window CT image, showing the main lung structures, associated with one mediastinal window CT image, highlighting the major mediastinal structures and lymph nodes. Figure 1.17 reveals the anatomical structures below the diaphragm.

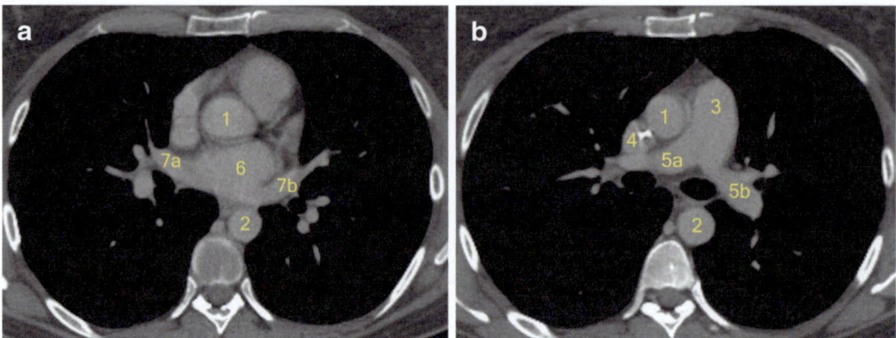

Fig. 1.11 Vascular tree. Axial chest CT images, mediastinal window, representing on the left (**a**) (1) Ascending aorta, (2) Descending aorta, (6) Left atrium, (7a) Pulmonary veins (right), (7b) Pulmonary veins (left); and on the right (**b**) (1) Ascending aorta, (2) Descending aorta, (3) Pulmonary trunk, (4) Superior vena cava, (5a) Right pulmonary artery, (5b) Left pulmonary artery

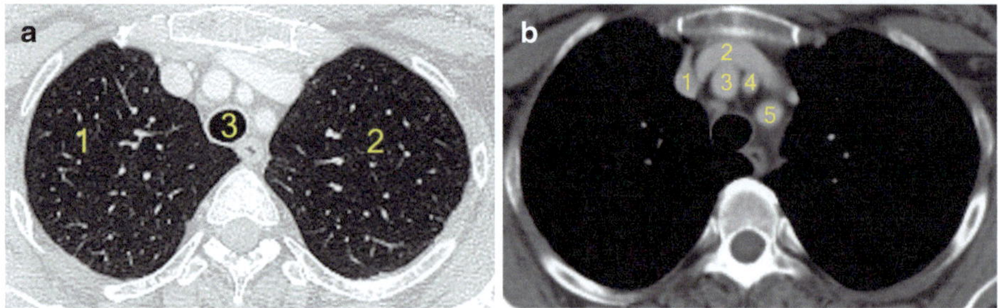

Fig. 1.12 Chest CT scan image, lung window (**a**): (1) Right upper lobe, (2) Left upper lobe, (3) Trachea. Chest CT scan image, mediastinal window (**b**): (1) Right brachiocephalic vein, (2) Left brachiocephalic vein, (3) Brachiocephalic artery, (4) Left common carotid, (5) Left subclavian artery

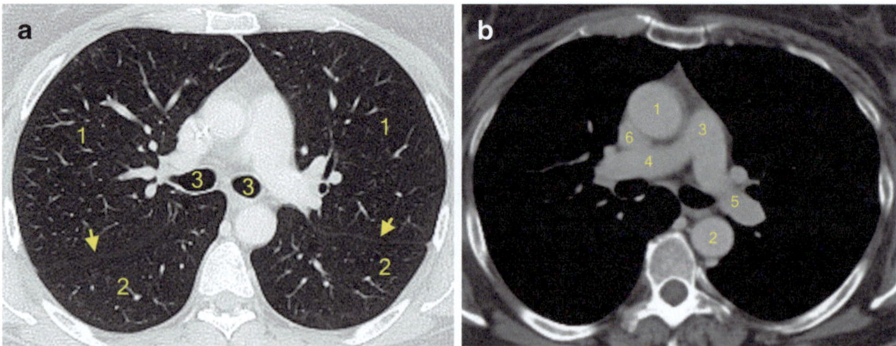

Fig. 1.13 Chest CT scan image, lung window (**a**): (1) Upper lobe, (2) Lower lobe, (3) Main bronchus (right/left), (Arrows) Major fissure. Chest CT scan image, mediastinal window (**b**): (1) Ascending aorta, (2) Descending aorta, (3) Pulmonary trunk, (4) Right pulmonary artery, (5) Left pulmonary artery, (6) Superior vena cava

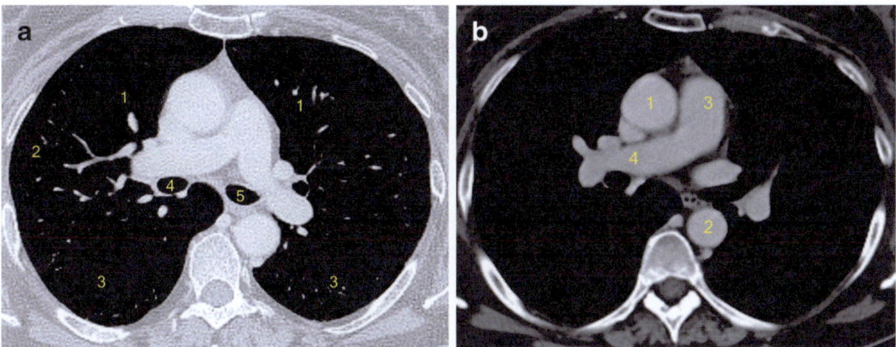

Fig. 1.14 Chest CT scan image, lung window (**a**): (1) Upper lobe, (2) Middle lobe, (3) Lower lobe, (4) Right main bronchus, (5) Left main bronchus. Chest CT scan image, mediastinal window (**b**): (1) Ascending aorta, (2) Descending aorta, (3) Pulmonary trunk, (4) Right pulmonary artery

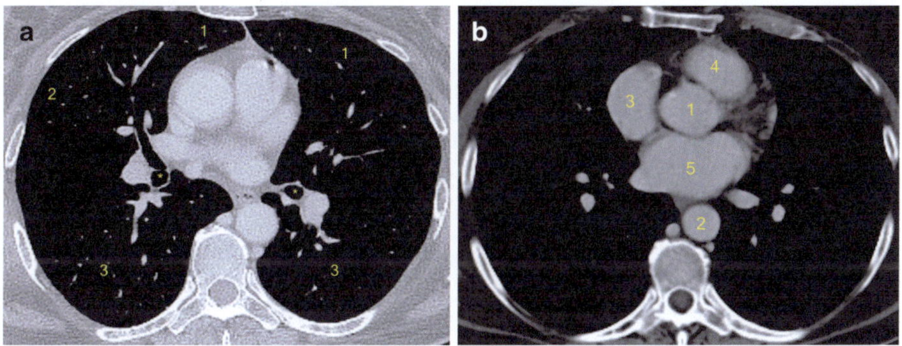

Fig. 1.15 Chest CT scan image, lung window (**a**): (1) Upper lobe, (2) Middle lobe, (3) Lower lobe, (∗) Lower lobe bronchus (right/left). Chest CT scan image, mediastinal window (**b**) (1) Ascending aorta, (2) Descending aorta, (3) Right atrium, (4) Right ventricle, (5) Left atrium

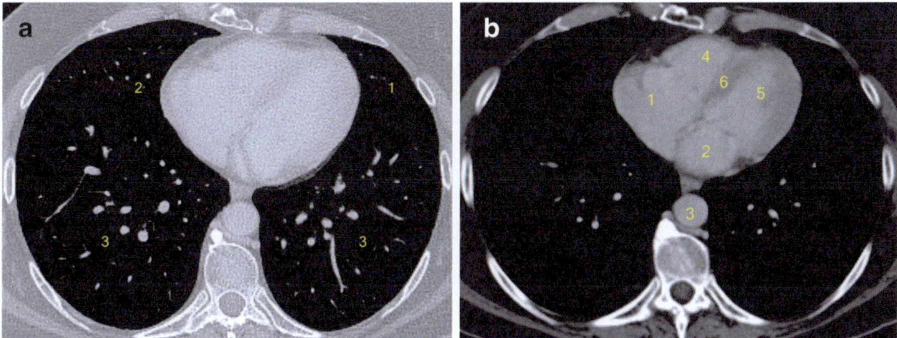

Fig. 1.16 Chest CT scan image, lung window (**a**): (1) Left upper lobe, (2) Middle lobe, (3) Lower lobe. Chest CT scan image, mediastinal window (**b**): (1) Right atrium, (2) Left atrium, (3) Descending aorta, (4) Right ventricle, (5) Left ventricle, (6) Interventricular septum

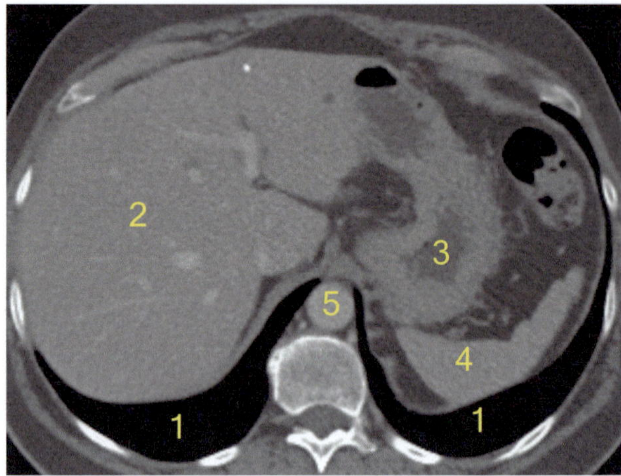

Fig. 1.17 (1) Lower lobe, (2) Liver, (3) Stomach, (4) Spleen, (5) Descending aorta

Suggested Readings

Ellis SM, Flower C. The WHO manual of diagnostic imaging: radiographic anatomy and interpretation of the chest and the pulmonary system. Geneva: World Health Organization; 2006.

El-Sherief, et al. International Association for the Study of Lung Cancer (IASLC) lymph node map: radiologic review with CT illustration. Radiographics. 2014;34:1680–91.

Gotway M. Netter's correlative imaging: cardiothoracic anatomy. 1st ed. Elsevier; 2013.

Moeller TB, Reif E. Pocket atlas of cross-sectional anatomy: computed tomography and magnetic resonance imaging, vol. 2. Thorax, abdomen, and pelvis. New York: Thieme Publishers; 1994.

Glossary

2

Isabella Ceravolo, Michele Anzidei,
and Cristina Marrocchio

The ability to identify a radiological sign and correlate it to a specific pathological condition is essential to refer the patient to a rapid diagnosis and a possible care in every clinical setting.

The field of thoracic radiology has developed a wide range of descriptions of signs, patterns, and metaphors to describe the anatomy and the main pathological processes, maybe more than any other radiological subspecialty. This small glossary is adapted and simplified on the basis of a much more comprehensive one, redacted by the Fleischner society; its intent is to clarify the vocabulary needed to describe the main diagnostic findings on CT scans. We will provide the most appropriate terms to describe an anatomical structure, an alteration, or a pathological pattern standing in correlation with information provided by clinicians and pathologists.

Even nowadays, terms such as "tree-in-bud sign" or "ground glass opacification" are used in reports without associating them to the correct pathological context and sometimes their meanings are confused; in many ways, not being able to express conclusions of a CT examination concisely, effectively and intelligibly, is as bad as neglecting radiological signs. A straightforward communication of the findings to both the patient and the clinician (with or without metaphors) is therefore as important as identifying them in the first place.

Basic Radiological Terminology

Density: this term is used in CT images. Hyperdense refers to structures with high attenuation (appearing whiter); hypodense refers to structure with low attenuation (appearing blacker).

I. Ceravolo · M. Anzidei (✉) · C. Marrocchio
Department of Radiological, Oncological and Pathological Sciences, Sapienza University of Rome, Rome, Italy

I. Carbone, M. Anzidei (eds.), *Thoracic Radiology*,
https://doi.org/10.1007/978-3-030-35765-8_2

Intensity: this term is used in MRI. Hyperintense refers to structures with high signal intensity (appearing brighter); hypointense refers to structure with decreased signal intensity (appearing darker).

Radiolucent and radiopaque: these terms refer to conventional radiographs. Radiolucent is used for structures with decreased density (=appearing black on a radiograph) that are structures that let the X-rays pass through them. Radiopaque refers to structures with high density (=appearing white on a radiograph) that are structures absorbing most of the X-rays.

Anatomy

Acinus

A pulmonary acinus is the structural unit of the lung. It is placed distal to the terminal bronchiole and contains the alveolar ducts and the alveoli. One lobule may contain 3 to 25 acini. Under normal conditions, acini cannot be visualized on imaging because of their small size; however, acinar arterioles may occasionally be identified in HRCT. The accumulation of pathological material within the acini can result in nodular opacities visible on chest X-ray or HRCT.

Aortopulmonary Window

The aortopulmonary window is a pleuromediastinal reflection that during fetal life is occupied by the ductus arteriosus.

Boundaries

- anterior: ascending aorta
- posterior: descending aorta
- cranial: aortic arc
- inferior: left pulmonary artery
- medial: ligamentum arteriosum
- lateral: pleura and left lung.

On a frontal radiograph, it is recognized as a focal concavity in the left mediastinal border below the aorta and above the left pulmonary artery. The aortopulmonary window is a common site of lymphadenopathy in a variety of neoplastic and inflammatory diseases.

Azygoesophageal Recess

The azygoesophageal recess is a prevertebral space where the edge of the right lower lobe extends between the heart and the vertebral column. Its margin forms a smooth arc convex to the left and its boundaries are:

- superior: azygos arch
- posterior: pleura anterior to the vertebral column
- medial: esophagus and adjacent structures
- inferior: right hemidiaphragm

On frontal chest X-ray, the recess is seen as a vertical stripe from the azygos arch to the right hemidiaphragm, running between the right lower lobe and the mediastinum. This space is best assessed on CT scans.

Bulla

A bulla is an air-space larger than 1 cm, demarcated by a thin wall not thicker than 1 mm. When inferior to 1 cm, the term bleb may be used. Bullae are usually present in an emphysematous lung, especially in paraseptal and centrilobular emphysema, and are commonly found in a subpleural location.

Bronchiole

Bronchioles are non-cartilage-containing airways. Distal to the conducting airways, there are the terminal bronchioles, from which the respiratory bronchioles originate. Distal to these are the alveolar ducts, whose walls are composed of alveoli that permit gas exchange. One respiratory bronchiole branches out into multiple alveolar ducts. Therefore, bronchioles are the transitional airways between the purely conducting airways and the alveolar ducts with the gas-exchanging alveoli. Bronchioles are not identifiable in healthy individuals because their wall is too thin. They become visible in inflammatory small-airways diseases, when they become thickened or plugged.

Bronchocentric

This term describes diseases centered on bronchovascular bundles, such as sarcoidosis, Kaposi sarcoma, and organizing pneumonia.

Centrilobular Region

The term centrilobular describes the central region of the secondary pulmonary lobule, which includes the area surrounding the centrilobular artery and centrilobular bronchiole. On CT scan, the centrilobular artery can be appreciated as a small dot-like or linear opacity in the center of a normal secondary pulmonary lobule, easier to identify in the subpleural area. Pathologies in this region can be tree-in-bud opacities, centrilobular nodules, centrilobular emphysema, or thickening/infiltration of the adjacent interstitium.

Fissure

A fissure is the infolding of the visceral pleura between two pulmonary lobes. On CT scans, they appear as regular lines with a thickness of 1 mm or less. The left lung has an oblique fissure; the right lung has two fissures: the minor (or horizontal) fissure and the major (or oblique) fissure. A very common anatomical variant are supernumerary fissures, which separate various segments within the same lobe. The azygos fissure, unlike the others, is formed by two layers each of visceral and parietal pleura, and delineates the azygos lobe, an anatomical variant present in 1% of the population.

Hilum

The lung hilum is the site on the medial aspect of the lung where the vessels and bronchi enter and leave the lung. On CT scans, the hilum is easy to find and the structures making it up (bronchi, arteries, veins, lymph nodes, nerves, and other tissues) can be well visualized at high resolutions.

Interstitium

The interstitium is the supporting connective tissue of the lung. It has three main subdivisions:

- the bronchovascular interstitium, surrounding and supporting the bronchi, arteries, veins, and lymphatics from the hilum to the respiratory bronchioles
- the parenchymal or acinar interstitium, interposed between the alveolar and capillaries basement membranes
- the subpleural connective tissue, contiguous with the interlobular septa

Lobe

The lobe is the principal division of the lung (three lobes on the right and two on the left). Each lobe is wrapped by the visceral pleura, except near the hilum.

Lobule

The lobule (or secondary pulmonary nodule) is the smallest structural unit of the lung bounded by connective tissue septa. It is a roughly polyhedral structure, 1–2 cm in size; the lobules in the peripheral regions of the lung are larger and more regular in shape, becoming smaller and more irregular in the central portions. Each SPL is constituted by 3–15 acini and 30–50 alveoli and is fed by a small centrilobular bronchiole and a small centrilobular artery. Venous and lymphatic drainage are in the surrounding connective tissue septa. The interlobular septa appear as thin structures on CT scans, but are usually hard to identify in a healthy lung.

Perilymphatic Distribution

Perilymphatic distribution indicates a pattern along the pulmonary lymphatic vessels, therefore along the bronchovascular tree, the interlobular septa, the pulmonary veins, and the pleura (alveoli do not have lymphatics). On CT scans, a pathological process has a perilymphatic distribution if it occurs in the perihilar, peribronchovascular, and centrilobular interstitium.

Perilobular Pattern

It refers to opacities or ground-glass involving the structures at the periphery of the secondary pulmonary lobule (i.e., interlobular septa, visceral pleura, and vessels).

Right Paratracheal Stripe

The right paratracheal stripe is a vertical, linear, soft-tissue opacity less than 4 mm in thickness that can be identified on a frontal chest X-ray. It represents the linear interface of the pleura of the upper lobe with the right border of the trachea and the mediastinal fat. It extends superoinferiorly for 3–4 cm, from the clavicles to the tracheobronchial angle at the level of the azygos arch. It is seen in 94% of adults. There are numerous pathologies that widens, deform, or obliterate this stripe including: paratracheal lymph node enlargement or pleural, tracheal, thyroid, and parathyroid diseases. It can also be hard to assess in non-pathological conditions such as in individuals with abundant mediastinal fat.

Segment

Bronchopulmonary segments are anatomically and functionally independent units within the lobes with an own ventilation (segment of the bronchus), vascular supply (branches of the pulmonary artery), and venous drainage. Each lobe can be composed of two to five segments.

Subpleural Curvilinear Line

A subpleural curvilinear line is a linear opacity 1–3 mm thick, parallel to and less than 1 cm from the pleural surface. It may indicate atelectasis, edema, or fibrosis.

Pathologic Processes

Air-Space

An air-space is the gas-containing part of the lung, excluding the conducting airways. It is a term used to specify the location of pathological alterations (air-space consolidation or nodules).

Air Trapping

Air trapping is a term referred to CT imaging indicating retention of air in the lungs distal to an obstruction, usually partial. An end-expiration CT scan can detect even small air trapping. At the end of expiration, as the lung becomes less expanded, the density of the lung parenchyma increases. Where air trapping is present, the increase in attenuation is less than the surrounding normal parenchyma and the volume does not decrease.

Atelectasis

Atelectasis is a reduced ventilation of a part or all of the pulmonary parenchyma. It appears on radiographs and CT as a decrease in volume, usually leading to an increase in opacity or density of the affected area. One of the most common causes of atelectasis is air reabsorption distal to an airway obstruction (obstructive atelectasis) but there are many mechanisms that may be involved (passive, compressive, adhesive, scarring, or dependent atelectasis). Atelectasis is often associated with shifts of the adjacent anatomical structures, such as fissures, hemidiaphragm, or mediastinum, towards the collapsed area. Based on its morphology, it can be classified as linear, round, or plate-like. Based on distribution, it can be lobar, segmental, or subsegmental.

Bronchiectasis

Bronchiectasis is permanent and irreversible, localized or diffuse, bronchial dilation usually resulting from chronic infections, proximal airway obstructions, or congenital abnormalities. Plain radiographs are relatively insensitive. In severe cases, they may appear as "tram-track" opacities or ring-shaped opacities, but they are difficult to appreciate. The typical CT appearance is a dilated bronchus, with a diameter larger than the accompanying artery (normally they are roughly of the same size), that is the signet-ring sign. Other findings can be lack of tapering of bronchi, and bronchi visible within 1 cm of the pleural surface. Bronchial wall thickening, mucoid impaction, and small-airways abnormalities are also commonly present. The three basic morphologic types of bronchiectasis are cylindrical, varicose, and cystic; different types can coexist.

Broncholith

A broncholith is a peribronchial calcified lymph node that erodes the bronchial wall and appears on CT scans as a calcified opacity within a bronchus, more often in the middle lobes. It often occurs secondary to histoplasma or M. tuberculosis infections. They may be asymptomatic or cause nonspecific symptoms.

Bronchiolitis

Bronchiolitis is an inflammation of the membranous and respiratory bronchioles. On CT scans, the characteristic sign is tree-in-bud opacities.

Bronchocele

A bronchocele is a dilated mucus-filled bronchus, usually caused by proximal obstruction. On chest X-rays, bronchocele appears as a tubular or branching Y- or V-shaped structure (finger in glove sign). The CT attenuation of the mucus is generally that of soft tissue but may be modified by its composition.

Cavity

A cavity is a gas-filled space seen as a low-attenuation area within a pulmonary consolidation, mass, or nodule. It sometimes contains a fluid level.

Cysts

A cyst is a round space, well-defined from the surrounding parenchyma, surrounded by an epithelial or fibrous wall of variable thickness (<2 mm), and containing air or—less commonly—fluid/solid material. Generally, they occur without associated pulmonary emphysema.

Honeycombing

Honeycombing describes a fibrotic pulmonary parenchyma replaced by numerous gaseous cysts in a honeycombing pattern, with total loss of acinar structure. The cysts range in size from few millimeters to several centimeters in diameter, have variable wall thicknesses, and are aligned with each other. On chest X-ray, ring-like opacities resembling bee honeycombs are visible. On CT scans, they appear as clusters of subpleural cysts with well-defined walls. Honeycombing is the late stage of many lung diseases; it is considered a specific sign of pulmonary fibrosis and is a key finding to diagnose usual interstitial pneumonia.

Interlobular Septal Thickening

On CT scans, it appears as a septal pattern. On chest X-ray, it appears as Kerley B lines, that are thin linear opacities of 1–2 cm at a 90° angle with respect to the surface of the parietal pleura near the lung base; they are typical in lymphangitic spread of lung cancer or pulmonary edema. It can also appear as Kerley A lines that are located in the upper lobes, are 2–6 mm long, and extend radially towards the hilum.

Lymphadenopathy

Lymphadenopathy is a broad term, usually used to describe an increase in size of a lymph node. The size of lymph nodes varies greatly depending on the anatomical site (e.g., inguinal lymph nodes are normally larger than mediastinal lymph nodes); therefore, a general cut-off value to distinguish a normal lymph node from a pathological one does not exist. Indicative thresholds can be used according to the anatomical region; nevertheless, size alone is not a reliable indicator of a lymph node pathology.

Mass

Term used to indicate any pulmonary, pleural, or mediastinal lesion greater than 3 cm in diameter.

Nodule

A nodule is a round or irregular opacity, well or poorly defined, maximum 3 cm in diameter. Nodules can be classified into micronodules, solid, part-solid, or non-solid nodules. A micronodule measures less than 3 mm. A non-solid nodule is a nodule with ground-glass density, which means that the underlying pulmonary structures (vessels, airways) can still be identified; a solid nodule is of homogeneous soft-tissue density and obscures the underlying lung parenchyma. A part-solid nodule consists of both solid tissue and ground-glass components.

Oligemia

Oligemia describes blood volume reduction, frequently regional but occasionally generalized.

Parenchymal Opacification

It is an area of the lung parenchyma with increased attenuation. The opacification can be a *consolidation*, that is a homogeneous increase in attenuation of the lung parenchyma that obscures the underlying pulmonary structures (vessels and airways). This occurs when the alveolar air is replaced. The opacification can also refer to an *area of ground-glass density*, which is an irregular, hazy opacity of the parenchyma in which the underlying pulmonary structures can still be identified. Ground-glass is caused by partial filling of air-spaces, interstitial thickening, partial collapse of alveoli, or increased capillary blood volume.

Pleural Plaque

Pleural plaques are acellular collagenous matrix deposits, sometimes with calcium salts inclusions appearing on CT as well-demarcated pleural thickenings, 1–5 cm in size. They more commonly affect the parietal diaphragmatic pleura or the pleura underneath the ribs. Pleural plaques are strongly associated to asbestos exposure and their extension correlates with the intensity of the chronic inhalation.

Pneumatocele

A pneumatocele is a gas-filled cystic space in the lung parenchyma surrounded by a proper wall. It may result from pneumonia or trauma, for a combination of parenchymal necrosis and check-valve airway obstruction. A pneumatocele may become secondarily infected, or it may rupture in the pleural space resulting in a pneumothorax.

Pseudocavity

A pseudocavity is a round or oval area of low attenuation within nodules, masses, or consolidations in the lung parenchyma. It usually measures less than 1 cm and does not have any boundary. It can represent normal parenchyma, normal or ectatic bronchi, or focal emphysema.

Pseudoplaque

A pseudoplaque is a lung opacity contiguous with the visceral pleura, formed by coalescent small nodules. It can appear similar to a pleural plaque. It is a common finding in sarcoidosis, silicosis, and pneumoconiosis due to carbon exposure.

Small-Airways Disease

This is a nonspecific term describing any pathological condition affecting the bronchioles. On CT scans, a small-airways disease is any alteration involving the airways with a diameter less than 2 mm and with the parietal thickness less than 0.5 mm. It can manifest as various patterns: mosaic attenuation, air trapping, centrilobular micronodules, tree-in-bud pattern, etc.

Patterns and Signs

Air Bronchogram

Generally, bronchi are not visible because they are thin-walled structures containing air and surrounded by air. When the parenchyma surrounding a bronchus becomes opaque and non-ventilated, the air-filled bronchus within it becomes visible and is called air bronchogram. This sign implies patency of proximal airways in an area of atelectatic or consolidated lung tissue (e.g., pneumonia), and it indicates the presence of an air-space disease.

Air Crescent Sign

When there is a cavity within the lung parenchyma, an air crescent describes a crescent-shaped collection of air, on CT or plain radiographs, that separates the wall of the cavity from an inner mass. The air crescent sign is often considered characteristic of either Aspergillus colonization of preexisting cavities or angioinvasive aspergillosis. However, the air crescent sign has also been reported in other conditions, including tuberculosis, Wegener granulomatosis, intracavitary hemorrhage, and lung cancer.

Crazy Paving Pattern

Crazy paving pattern describes the combination of a septal pattern with ground-glass opacities. Surrounding areas of healthy parenchyma are visible. It was initially described in patients with alveolar proteinosis, but other lung pathologies that simultaneously involve both interstitial and air-spaces may cause this pattern as well.

Halo Sign

On CT scans, the halo sign is a ground-glass opacity surrounding a nodule or mass. This sign is not specific for a single pathology. It may be secondary to hemorrhage (e.g., in angioinvasive aspergillosis) or to pulmonary infiltration by a carcinoma (e.g., adenocarcinoma).

A **reversed halo sign** is a ground-glass opacity surrounded by crescent-shaped or ring-shaped consolidated parenchyma. An extremely rare finding, it has been reported in cryptogenic organizing pneumonia and paracoccidioidomycosis.

Mosaic Attenuation Pattern

Mosaic attenuation pattern describes the presence of regions with different attenuations within the lung parenchyma. The pathological parenchyma can be either the regions with higher attenuation or the regions with lower attenuations, depending on the underlying pathological process; this is not always an easy distinction. The three main causes of this pattern are: interstitial diseases (in which regions with higher attenuation are the pathological ones, representing the areas where the interstitium is involved); small-airways obstruction (in which regions with lower attenuation are the pathological ones, representing regions with air trapping. This appearance may be better appreciated on expiratory HRCT); oligemia or mosaic perfusion patterns (in which regions with lower attenuation are the pathological ones, representing regions with decreased blood-flow).

Nodular Pattern

The nodular pattern is characterized by nodules less than 1 cm in size that, according to their distribution, can be classified as random, miliary, centrilobular, or perilymphatic. On chest X-ray, nodules are small (2–10 mm) spread ubiquitously in the pulmonary parenchyma.

Reticular Pattern

On CT scans, a reticular pattern is characterized by small and numerous intralobular linear opacities. As the disease progresses, interlobular septal thickening and traction bronchiectasis are also observed.

Reticulonodular Pattern

This pattern is a combination of nodular and reticular patterns, with the presence of micronodules and reticular elements.

Septal Pattern

This pattern is due to the interlobular septal thickening. It appears as short lines in the periphery of the lung that arrive to the pleura. Based on the appearance of the septa, it can be classified as smooth, nodular, or irregular.

Signet-Ring Sign

Usually, a bronchus and its accompanying vessel should be roughly of the same size. Signet-ring sign describes a ring-shaped opacity, where the ring itself represents the walls of a dilated bronchus and the signet is the small vessel adjacent to it. On CT scans, it is the typical sign of bronchiectasis.

Silhouette Sign

When on plain radiographs, structures of similar attenuations overlap, the normal anatomical soft-tissue contours, such as the borders of the heart or the outline of the diaphragm, become unrecognizable. This may occur in pathological conditions, such as a consolidations, atelectasis, or pleural fluid accumulation, but is not always indicative of a disease process (e.g., absence of the right margin of the heart can be present in subjects with pectus excavatum, or sometimes in healthy subjects).

Tree-in-bud (TIB) Pattern

This CT sign describes bronchiolar ramifications originating from a single stalk associated with small centrilobular nodules that resembles a tree-in-bud. It occurs secondary to centrilobular thickening and endo- and peri-bronchiolar deposition of compact mucus, inflammation, and/or fibrosis. This finding is not visible on plain radiographs but is best seen with HRCT; usually, it is more prominent in the peripheral portions of the lung parenchyma. This pattern is common in panbronchiolitis, endobronchial spread of mycobacterial infection or cystic fibrosis but it may be recognized in many lung diseases.

Suggested Readings

Austin JH, et al. Glossary of terms for CT of the lungs: recommendations of the Nomenclature Committee of the Fleischner Society. Radiology. 1996;200(2):327–31.

Hall FM. Fleischner Society glossary of terms: infiltrates. Radiology. 2008;248(3):1083.

Hansell DM, et al. Fleischner Society: glossary of terms for thoracic imaging. Radiology. 2008;246(3):697–722.

Langlotz CP. The completeness of existing lexicons for representing radiology report information. J Digit Imaging. 2002;15(Suppl 1):201–5.

3 Introduction to Chest X-Ray Interpretation

Vincenzo Noce and Rosa Maria Ammendola

A chest radiograph—or chest X-ray (CXR)—is the most commonly requested first-line examination for the diagnosis of numerous clinical scenarios thanks to the widespread availability, low radiation doses, and modest costs. CXRs are optimal to confirm clinical suspicions based on specific signs and symptoms; however, without a proper diagnostic suspicion beforehand, its accuracy drops drastically. CXRs also play a decisive role in the intensive care unit, being fundamental for a quick assessment of patient conditions and to verify the correct placement of intensive-care devices (venous catheters, cannulas for ventilation, etc.).

Technical Considerations

CXRs can be acquired in many projections; the standard protocol includes a posteroanterior (PA) and a lateral (LL) projection (Fig. 3.1a, b). To optimize quality, all projections should be acquired at full inspiration with the patient standing at a distance of 180 cm from the X-ray source.

The anteroposterior (AP) projection can be obtained with a supine, semi-recumbent or sitting patient depending on the patient's compliance during the exam. The main disadvantage of this projection is creating excessive distortion, thus falsely enlarging the cardiac silhouette which may in itself lead to incorrect diagnoses or cover pathological processes within the overshadowed lung fields (Fig. 3.1c). Lateral projections allow for a more complete exploration of mediastinal structures (particularly the hila) and the pulmonic recesses not visible on the PA projection; it can also be used as a confirmation and for three-dimensional localization of the findings observed on a PA radiograph.

V. Noce · R. M. Ammendola (✉)
Department of Radiological, Oncological and Pathological Sciences, Sapienza University of Rome, Rome, Italy

I. Carbone, M. Anzidei (eds.), *Thoracic Radiology*,
https://doi.org/10.1007/978-3-030-35765-8_3

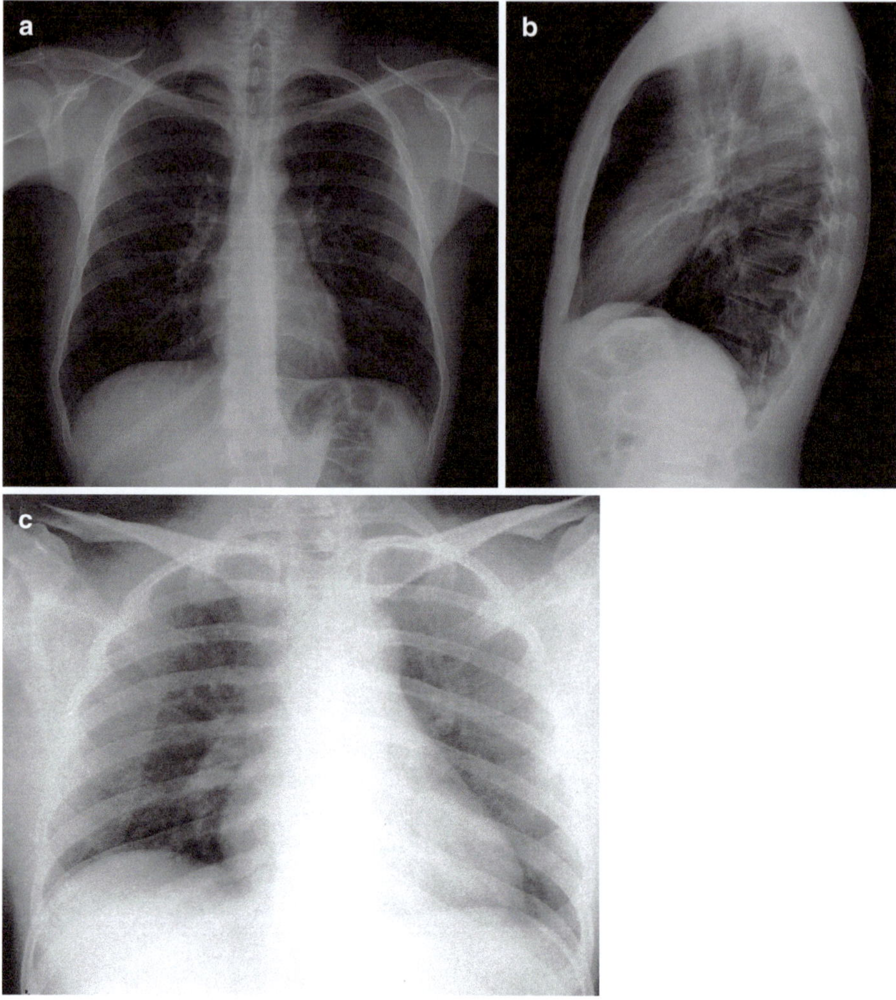

Fig. 3.1 (**a**) Standard posteroanterior projection. (**b**) Standard lateral projection. (**c**) Anteroposterior projection obtained with a portable device at the patient's bed

Some other projections not included in the standard exam are as follows:

- Expiratory view, for better visualization of pneumothorax
- Apical view, obtained by directing the X-ray beam superoinferiorly to have a better representation of the apical regions
- Oblique projection, obtained by orienting the patient at 45° with respect to the radiant beam, in order to study the sternum and the lateral side of costal arches

The technical adequacy of a standard X-ray examination is evaluated on the PA radiograph using the parameters summarized in the panel in Fig. 3.2.

b

Technical Adequacy of Chest x-ray	
Volume included in the radiograph	It should include from the lung apices to the constophrenic angles
Rotation	Medial ends of the clavicles should be simmetric to the vertebrae
Penetration	Evaluate the region behind the heart: the left hemidiaphragm and the vertebrae should be visible
Inspiration	The anterior costal arches should be visible from the first to the sixth rib

Fig. 3.2 Adequacy parameters (**b**) in the posteroanterior projection of the chest X-rays (**a**)

Anatomy of a Chest Radiograph

The two-dimensional image obtained with a CXR includes all structures contained within the irradiated volume superimposed on each other; these project differently on an image based on their position with respect to the incident X-rays. Hence, the anatomical information resulting from CXRs is "indirect," as opposed to the volumetric acquisition obtained with a CT scan. Nevertheless, many anatomical structures can still be detected and examined with radiography:

Large Airways

The trachea, carina, and main bronchi are visible as median radiolucent structures. The right main bronchus has a cranio-caudal orientation, while the left one describes a steeper angle towards the hilum.

Hilar Structures

The hila contain the main bronchi and the pulmonary vessels; lymph nodes should not be visible in a normal chest. Characteristically, the right hilum is more caudal than the left one and the arterial vessel is anterior to the main right bronchus. The left pulmonary artery is superior to the left bronchus and appears as an arch whose concavity is directed anteroinferiorly on lateral projections. Together with the aortic arch, it defines the aortopulmonary window. The inferior lobar branches of the pulmonary arteries should be visible as two fingers pointing towards the hemidiaphragm (Fig. 3.3).

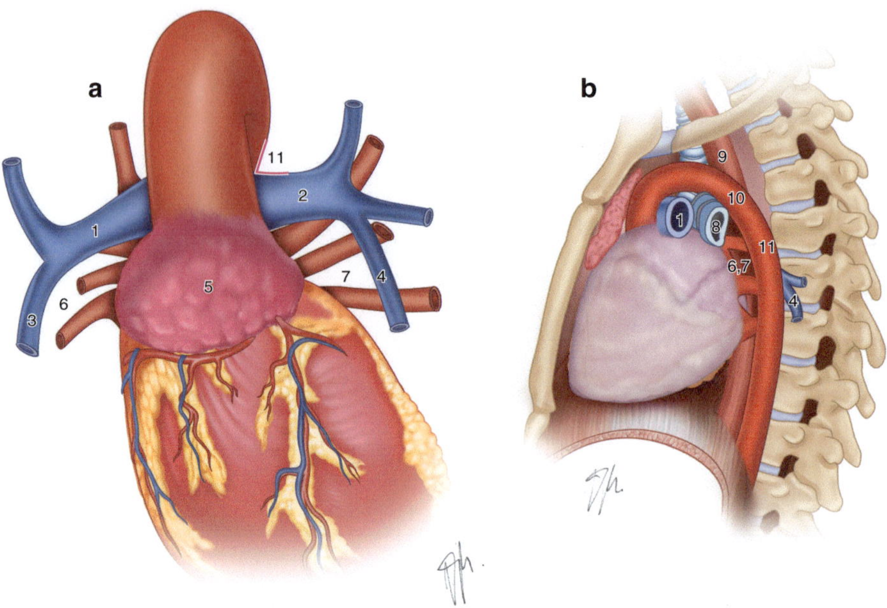

Fig. 3.3 Diagram of the main hilar structures in the PA (**a**) and LL (**b**) projections: (1) Right pulmonary artery, (2) Left pulmonary artery, (3) Right lower lobar pulmonary artery, (4) Left lower lobar pulmonary artery, (5) Right atrium, (6) Right pulmonary veins, (7) Left pulmonary veins, (8) Right main bronchus, (9) Trachea, (10) Aortic arch, (11) Aortopulmonary window

Mediastinum

The heart and main vessels are within the middle mediastinum, which is between the anterior (containing the thymus and mammary vessels) and posterior (containing the esophagus, descending aorta, azygos, and hemiazygos veins) mediastinum.

On PA projections, we can recognize five mediastinal arches, two on the right and three on the left side. Moreover, we can identify some lines which must always be examined in any chest X-ray because they might be the only visible alteration caused by an underlying pathology (Fig. 3.4).

The azygoesophageal line on the right and the paraaortic line on the left define the posteroinferior mediastinal space that may be involved in many pathological processes (hiatal hernia, esophageal or neurogenic neoplasms, lymphadenopathies).

The aortopulmonary window is a pleuromediastinal reflection that is occupied by the ductus arteriosus during fetal life. Straight or concave towards the lung, it can be easily identified on a PA projection and in a normal chest exam. If altered, it is often a sign of pathology in the anterosuperior mediastinum (lymphadenopathies, thymoma, etc.).

The right paratracheal stripe follows the right side of the trachea and is another useful reference point for studying the mediastinum; in a normal chest it must not exceed 3 mm in width.

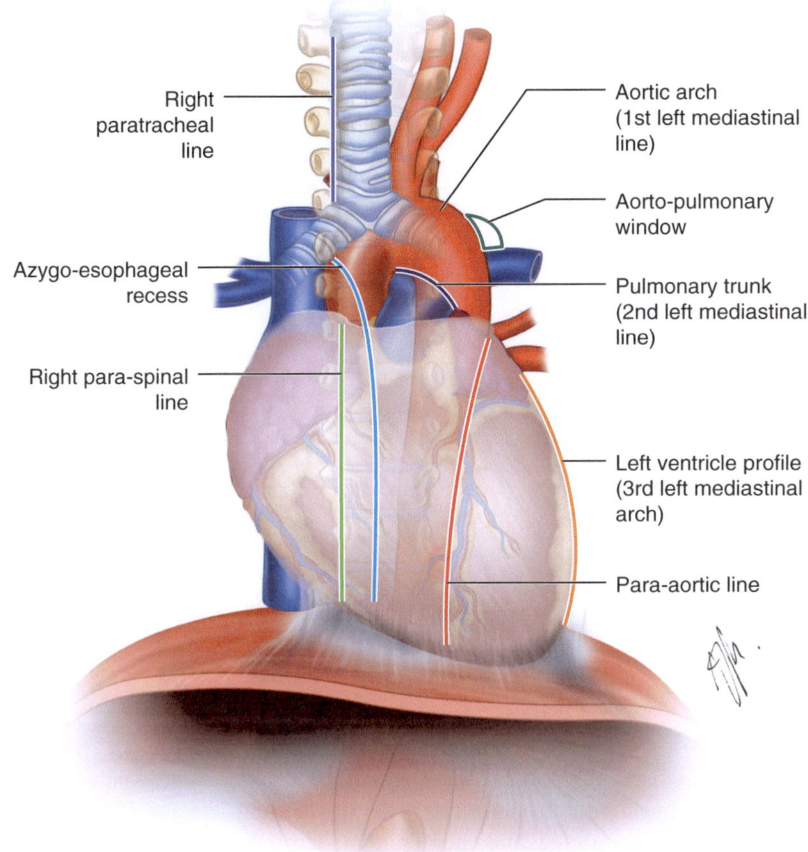

Fig. 3.4 Diagram of the main mediastinal contours

The paraspinal lines run along both sides of the dorsal vertebral column; often, only the right is visible and serves as reference for pathologies originating from the vertebrae.

Lung Parenchyma

To study the lung parenchyma on a chest X-ray, it should be divided into three regions (upper, middle, and lower lungs—Fig. 3.5), and their symmetry should be evaluated in terms of density and morphology. To locate the pathological processes within the lobes, both the PA and lateral projections must be correlated.

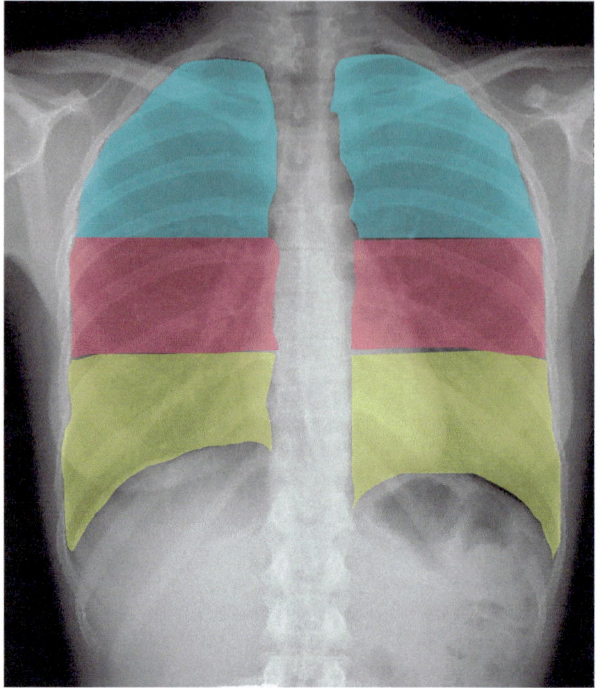

Fig. 3.5 Schematic representation of the division of the lung parenchyma in three regions. When assessing the lung parenchyma, the density of each region should be compared

Pleura

The parietal and visceral pleura are 0.2–0.4 mm thick and thus not visible on a standard CXR in physiological conditions (nor on a multidetector CT scan, being beyond its spatial resolution). The lateral and posterior costophrenic angles and the lung apices are the anatomical structures that are to be evaluated when studying the pleural space on a chest X-ray.

Hemidiaphragms

Normally, the diaphragm is 2–3 mm thick and not visible on a CXR. The right hemidiaphragm is more cranial than the contralateral. The left one can be pointed out by the presence of air in the fundus of the stomach ("gastric bubble"), while its contours disappear anteriorly in the lateral projection due to the heart shadow. Both hemidiaphragms form lateral and posterior costophrenic angles with the chest wall.

Heart and Pericardium

Cardiac size is usually evaluated by measuring the cardiothoracic ratio, which is less than 0.5 in physiological conditions, i.e., the heart should be less than half the

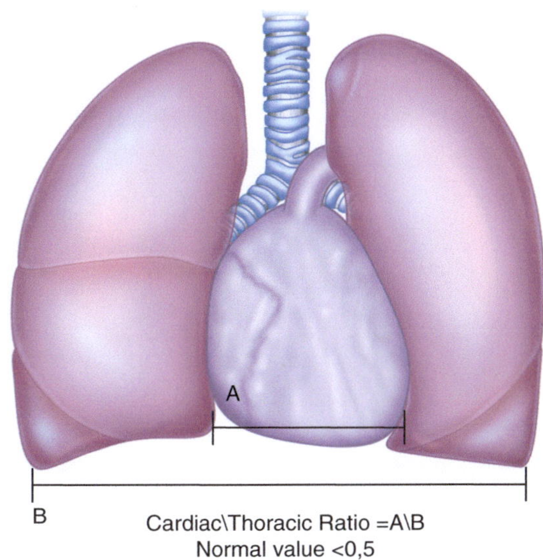

Fig. 3.6 Schematic representation of the calculation of the cardiothoracic ratio

side-to-side size of the thorax (Fig. 3.6). When studying the cardiac chambers on a CXR it is important to consider that the left ventricle and the right atrium are best examined on the frontal projection, while the right ventricle and the left atrium should be evaluated on the lateral projection. Normally, the pericardium cannot be seen on CXRs; when there is a significant pericardial effusion, the cardiac silhouette is enlarged but there are no specific signs that can be found on a radiograph.

Common Pathological Findings on Chest X-Rays

Pleural Pathology

A pneumothorax (PNX) is the finding on a chest radiograph with the most important immediate clinical impact. It is defined by the presence of air within the pleural space and is most commonly caused by thoracic traumas with rib fractures or spontaneous rupture of emphysematous bullae. Typically, it can be recognized by a radiolucent band variable in size within the pleura, lacking the normal pulmonary vasculature and often marked by a radiopaque line that represents the visceral pleura (Fig. 3.7). If the mediastinal structures are shifted away, it indicates a tension pneumothorax, i.e., a medical emergency in which a pneumothorax is enlarged and worsened with each respiratory act. When the patient is supine, it is possible to appreciate the pneumothorax in the costophrenic angles (deep sulcus sign, Fig. 3.7).

Significant pleural effusions (more than 2 L) characteristically appear as an opacification with an inferiorly concave meniscus shape (Damoiseau-Ellis line), a contralateral shift of the mediastinal structures and no volume loss in the hemithorax. With smaller amounts of fluid the costophrenic angles are blunted (Fig. 3.8).

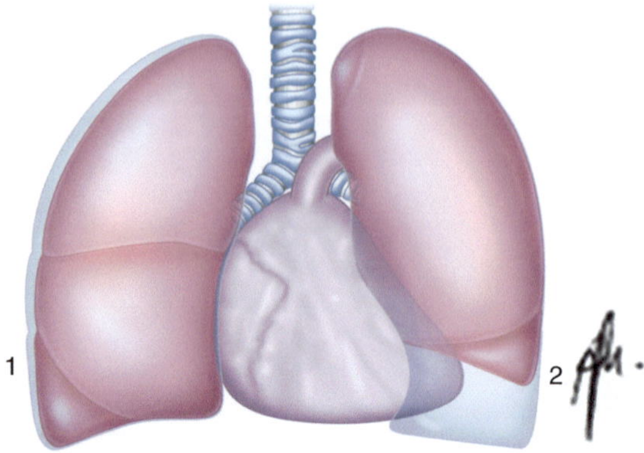

Fig. 3.7 Schematic representation of pneumothorax appearance in a standing (1) and a supine (2) patient

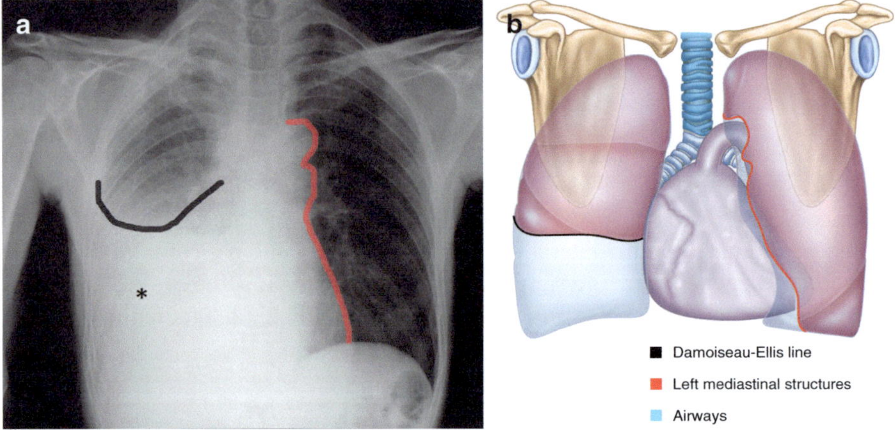

Fig. 3.8 Significant pleural effusion (∗) with the typical Damoiseau-Ellis line (*black line*) (**a**, **b**). Note that the left mediastinal structures (*red line*) are essentially not shifted because of associated atelectasis (**a**, **b**)

Pleural thickening can have numerous causes. If bilateral and involving the diaphragmatic pleura it may be due to asbestosis; if unilateral, the cause is tuberculosis, empyema, or hemorrhage. A single focal pleural thickening must always arise suspicion of pleural cancer.

Parenchymal Pathology

Parenchymal pathologies can be classified into five different patterns: consolidation, atelectasis, radiolucency, interstitiopathy, nodule/mass (Fig. 3.9).

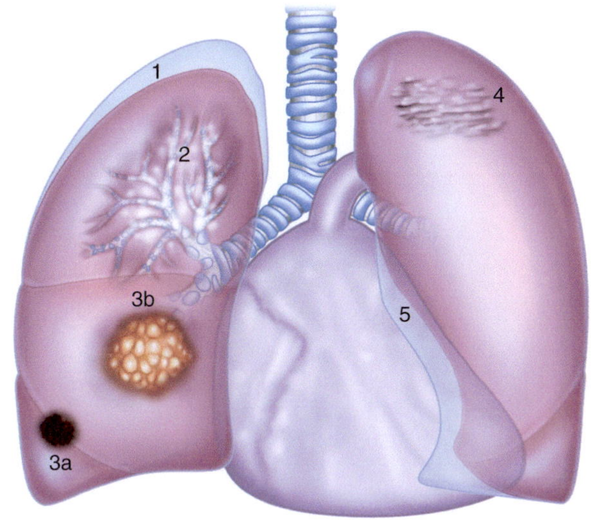

Fig. 3.9 Schematic representation of parenchymal lung disease patterns on chest X-rays: (1) Pneumothorax, (2) Consolidation, (3a) Nodule, (3b) Mass, (4) Interstitiopathy, (5) Atelectasis

Consolidation is by definition an area of opacification with irregular margins that respects the lobar boundaries and does not result in a significant loss of volume. It is caused by the replacement of the alveolar air with denser substances (blood, exudate, cells). In lobar pneumonia it is possible to visualize the small airways within the consolidated area (air bronchogram sign). In acute pulmonary edema the consolidations are bilateral, with perihilar confluence and associated with bilateral pleural effusion.

Nodules and masses are focal areas of radiopacity with well-defined margins; by definition, they are called nodules if they are less than 3 cm in size, and masses when larger than that.

Studying interstitiopathies on CXRs is very complex and often they are not discernible even when the clinical presentation is evident. The predominant patterns are the reticular and micronodular ones, which may sometimes overlap.

Atelectasis is the collapse of lung parenchyma caused by bronchial occlusion (neoplasia, mucus plugs, etc.). It appears as an opacification with well-defined margins, devoid of air bronchograms, with loss of volume and ipsilateral shift of mediastinal structures.

Suggested Readings

Gibbs JM, et al. Lines and stripes: where did they go? From conventional radiography to CT. Radiographics. 2007;27:33–48.

de Lacey et al. The chest X-ray: a survival guide. Saunders Elsevier, 2008.

Reed JC. Chest radiology plain film patterns and differential diagnoses. 6th Edition, Mosby, 2010.

Webb R, Higgins C. Thoracic imaging: pulmonary and cardiovascular radiology. 3rd Edition, Lippincott Williams, 2016.

Pulmonary Nodules: Identification and Risk Assessment

4

Carola Palla and Andrea Porfiri

A pulmonary nodule is defined as a spherical, rounded, or irregularly shaped and more or less defined parenchymal opacity with a diameter of up to 3 cm. Incidental, newly identified nodules of indeterminate (non-fibrocalcific) composition are a relatively common finding (8–51% prevalence on CT scans). In 96% of cases, multiple nodules are detected with a diameter of less than 10 mm; of these, up to 72% are smaller than 5 mm. Their malignancy rate is relatively low (1–12%, as reported). The proper management of incidental nodules is of particular importance and interest in thoracic radiology, as the early identification of malignant lesions benefits from curative surgical treatment and could help avoid invasive procedures in patients with benign lesions.

Maximum Intensity Projections (MIP) reconstructions significantly increase the sensitivity of lung nodule detection compared to the conventional technique (Fig. 4.1), particularly for nodules smaller than 5 mm.

Managing the Incidental Finding of an Indeterminate Pulmonary Nodule

The incidental finding of an indeterminate pulmonary nodule can be dealt with in different ways:

- Ignore the finding
- Schedule a follow-up CT scan
- Schedule a contrast-enhanced CT or PET-CT
- Perform a biopsy (fine needle aspiration or core biopsy)
- Perform surgery (open or video-assisted thoracoscopic surgery)

C. Palla (✉) · A. Porfiri
Department of Radiological, Oncological and Pathological Sciences, Sapienza University of Rome, Rome, Italy

I. Carbone, M. Anzidei (eds.), *Thoracic Radiology*,
https://doi.org/10.1007/978-3-030-35765-8_4

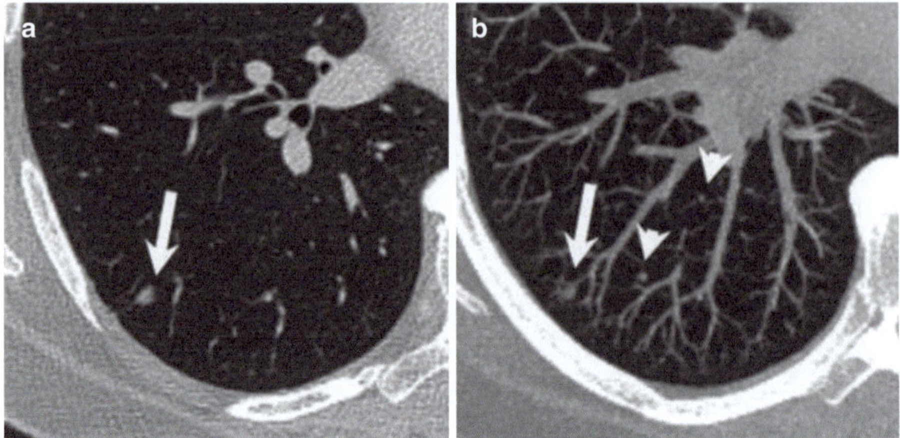

Fig. 4.1 Maximum Intensity Projections (MIP) reconstructions increase the detection of pulmonary nodules. (**a**) 1 mm standard axial image allows to identify a 5 mm nodule (*arrow*). (**b**) 20 mm axial MIP shows the presence of more nodules (*arrowheads*)

The choice of the most appropriate option is based on a careful evaluation of a patient's pre-test risk factors and the morphological characteristics of the nodule.

There are several risk factors for lung cancer, including: cigarette smoking, age, exposure to carcinogens (radon, asbestos, uranium), pulmonary fibrosis, a family history of cancer, or any previous neoplastic disease. Based on these risk factors, two categories of patients arise:

- High risk: cigarette smoking (risk increased 10–35 times), age >40 years, family history of cancer, previous neoplastic diseases
- Low risk: minimal or no smoking habit, age <40 years, no other known risk factors

The morphological characteristics to be evaluated to recognize malignancy include:

1. **Size**: There is strong evidence that the likelihood of a nodule to become malignant increases with its dimensions: nodules of <4 mm have a <1% probability of malignancy, while nodules of >8 mm have a >25% chance of being cancerous.
2. **Morphology—Shape—Position**: a polygonal or ovoid nodule, located peripherally or adjacent to the pleura, has a high probability of being benign (Fig. 4.2a). If located in the upper lobes, on the other hand, it is associated with a greater likelihood of malignancy. Nodules with regular margins have a prevalence of malignancy around 20–30% (Fig. 4.2a); this value increases to 33–100% in lesions with lobular, irregular, or spiky margins (Fig. 4.2b).
3. **Density**: Nodules can appear solid, with ground glass opacity (GGO) (Fig. 4.3b), or mixed (mixed ground glass opacity, mGGO) when they are not solid

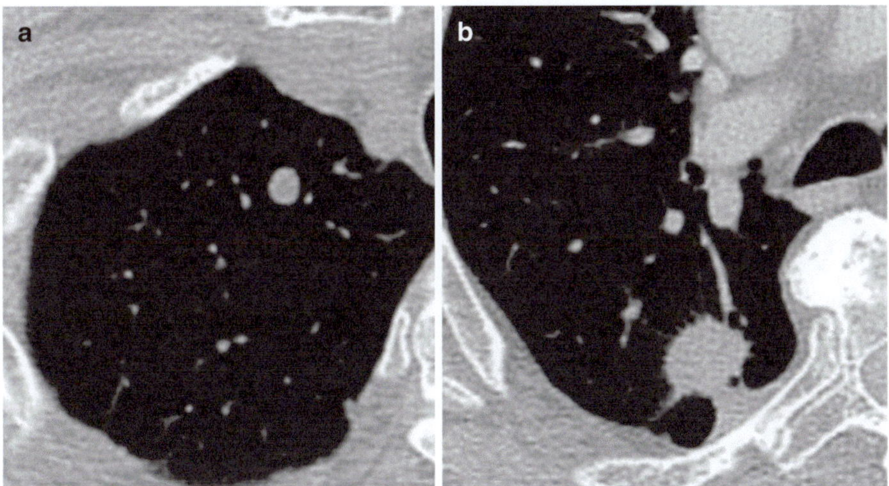

Fig. 4.2 (**a**) Benign solid nodule, ovoid, adjacent to the pleura, with regular margins, (**b**) Malignant solid nodule located in the right upper lobe with irregular margins

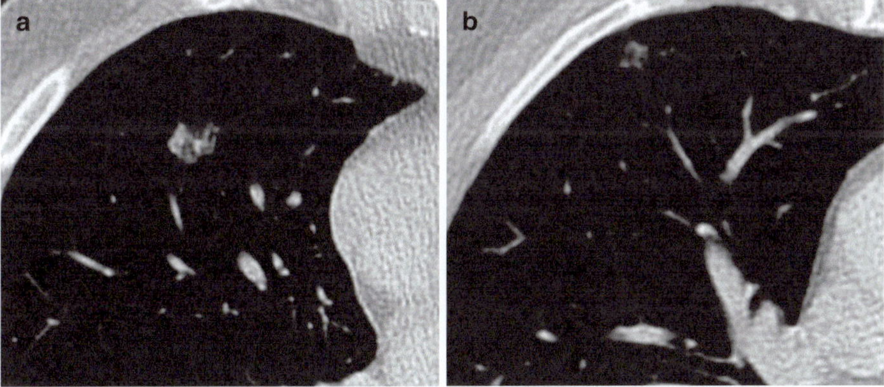

Fig. 4.3 (**a**) Mixed nodule, (**b**) Ground glass nodule

throughout (Fig. 4.3a). Partially solid or mixed nodules are more often regarded as malignant or potentially malignant lesions, including pre-invasive or early-invasive adenocarcinoma (previously described as bronchioalveolar adenocarcinoma or BAC), atypical adenomatous hyperplasia and, less frequently, local inflammatory or infectious disease processes or focal fibrosis. The prevalence of malignancy in these nodules varies with their composition, being 63%, 18%, and 7% in a mixed, non-solid, and fully solid nodule, respectively.

4. **Growth**: When malignant, the volume doubling time (VDT) of solid nodules is approximately 149 days (Fig. 4.4) Keeping the future follow-up in mind, always consider that malignant nodules grow faster in smokers than in non-smokers

The VDT of non-solid nodules is usually longer, with an average of 813 days (Fig. 4.5).

Finally, mixed nodules grow at an intermediate rate of about 457 days (Fig. 4.6).

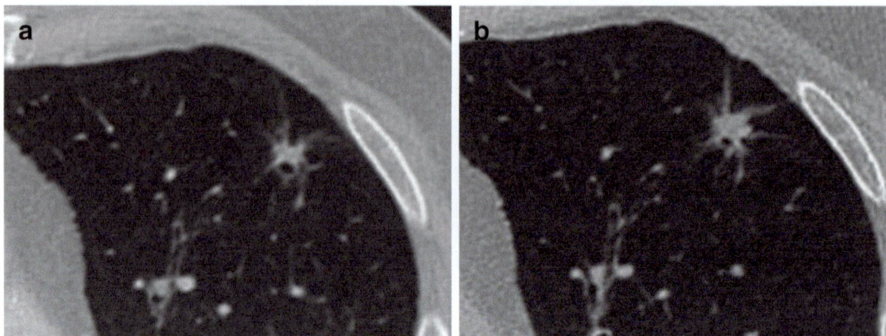

Fig. 4.4 Solid nodule. (**a**) Nodule when first observed, (**b**) Follow-up CT at 10 months. The nodule has grown

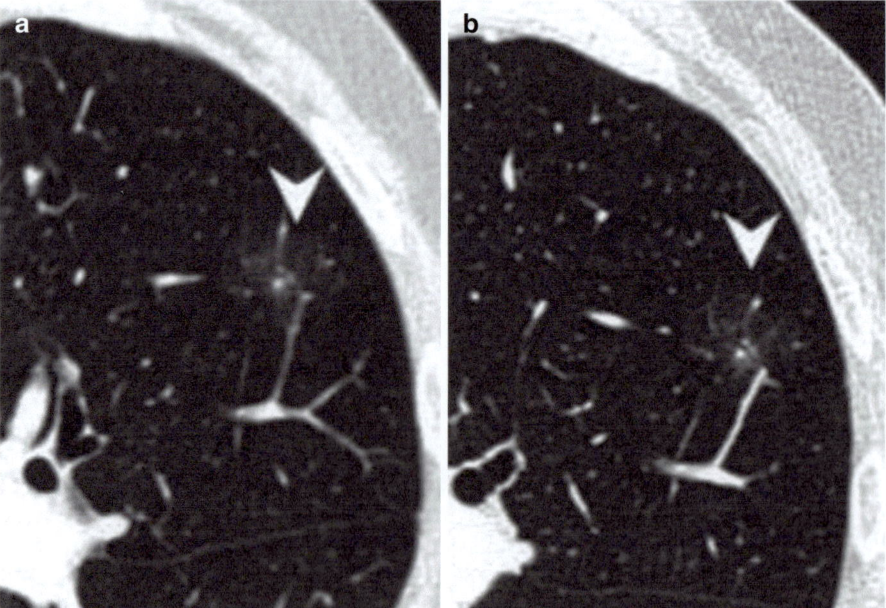

Fig. 4.5 Non-solid nodule exhibiting slow growth rate (*arrowhead*). (**a**) Nodule when first detected, (**b**) Follow-up after 6 months, (**c**) Follow-up after 12 months, with slow growth rate. Diagnostic study with fine needle aspiration biopsy revealed atypical adenomatous hyperplasia with nests of bronchioalveolar carcinoma cells

Fig. 4.5 (continued)

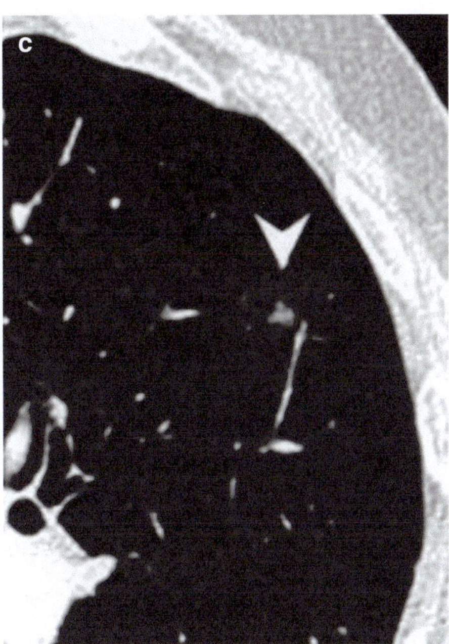

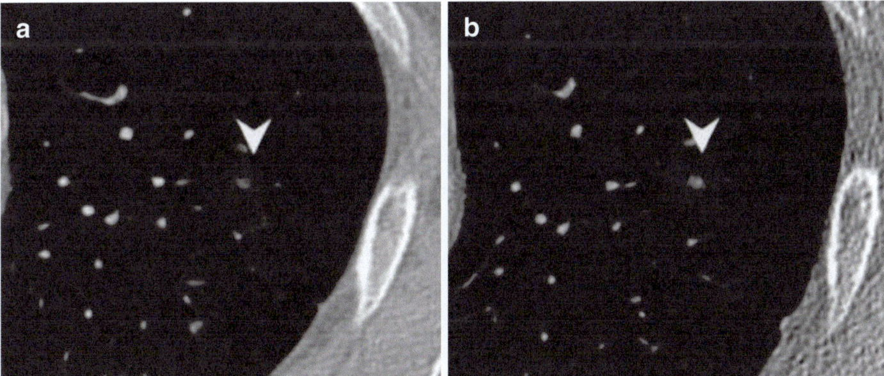

Fig. 4.6 Mixed nodule (*arrowhead*). (**a**) Nodule when first observed, (**b**) 10-month follow-up: both the size and the solid component have increased

Guidelines for the Management of Pulmonary Nodules

These guidelines are intended for adults older than 35 years (as lung cancer is rare in younger patients) without known primary cancers (and without any risk for metastases) in which an incidental finding of a pulmonary nodule is made. Table 4.1 gives an easy overview with simple cut-offs:

The unvarying size and morphology of a solid nodule at 2-year follow-up confirm its benignity with no need of further diagnostic tests; any occurring growth requires a histological diagnosis, except when specific clinical contraindications are present.

Special Considerations

1. *Patients with a history of or suspected cancer*: in case the primary tumor is known to be a possible cause of lung metastases, follow-up should be performed according to the guidelines for the primary neoplasia.
2. *Young patients*: in patients younger than 35 years, lung cancer is very rare and the risks for radiation exposure are higher. If there is no diagnosis of cancer, the follow-up of small incidental nodules with further CTs is not recommended. In these cases, a single low-dose CT follow-up within 6–12 months is considered more appropriate.
3. *Patients with fever of unknown origin*: sometimes, a lung nodule is an inflammatory or infectious focus. In these cases, consider a short-distance follow-up or a different diagnostic approach (bronchoscopy with bronchial lavage).

Non-solid or Partially Solid (Mixed) Lung Nodules

Non-solid nodules are areas of opacity with or without well-defined margins, through which normal lung parenchyma, vessels, and airways can be recognized. They can be benign (inflammatory), premalignant (atypical adenomatous hyperplasia or in situ adenocarcinoma), or malignant lesions (minimally invasive or invasive adenocarcinoma).

Due to long VDTs, a 2-year follow-up does not exclude malignancy. However, the aggressiveness of a lesion is of no certain prognostic value and may never become significant during the patient's life. Some recommendations are:

- Size and morphology are equally important when deciding about correct management.
- Mixed lesions should not be disbanded as "inflammatory outcomes" or "non-specific lesions." They require proper diagnostic intervention.
- As non-solid nodules grow more slowly, they should be studied with greater caution and a longer time interval between follow-up scans is desirable. The management for non-solid or partially solid lung nodules described by the 2017 Fleischner Society guidelines takes into account their size, number, and morphology, differentiating pure ground glass nodules from ground glass nodules with a solid component (Table 4.1).

Interestingly, there is no clear-cut difference in recommendations for smoking and non-smoking patients, contrary to solid nodules; this is partly due to the increase in incidence of adenocarcinoma in young and non-smoking individuals.

Table 4.1 Management of incidental pulmonary nodules (solid and non-solid)

Solid nodules				
	Single nodule		**Multiple nodules**	
	(<6 mm warrant no routine follow-up)	*(consider 12-month follow-up with suspicious morphology or upper lobe location)*	*Use most suspicious nodule as guide*	
Risk Size	**Low**	**High**	**Low**	**High**
<6 mm (<100 mm^2)	No routine follow-up	Optional CT at 12 months	No routine follow-up	Optional CT at 12 months
6–8 mm (100–250 mm^2)	CT at 6–12 months, consider CT after another 18–24 months	CT at 6–12 months, then CT after another 18–24 months	CT at 3–6 months, consider CT after another 18–24 months	CT at 3–6 months, then CT after another 18–24 months
>8 mm (>250 mm^2)	Consider CT at 3 months, PET/CT, or tissue sampling	Consider CT at 3 months, PET/CT, or tissue sampling	CT at 3–6 months, consider CT after another 18–24 months	CT at 3–6 months, then CT after another 18–24 months
Subsolid nodules				
Appearance Size	**Single, ground glass**	**Single, part solid**	**Multiple**	
<6 mm (<100 mm^2)	No routine follow-up	No routine follow-up	CT at 3–6 months. If stable, CT after another 2 and 4 years	
≥6 mm (100–250 mm^2)	CT at 6–12 months to confirm persistence, then CT every 2 years until 5 years	CT at 3–6 months to confirm persistence, if unchanged and solid component remains <6 mm, annual CT should be performed for 5 years	CT at 3–6 months; subsequent management based on the most suspicious nodule(s)	

Adapted from Guidelines for Management of Incidental Pulmonary Nodules Detected on CT Images: From the Fleischner Society 2017, MacMahon et al.

When a patient has a negative history of current or previous malignancy and no inflammatory, infectious or granulomatous disease processes are afoot, the management of multiple pulmonary nodules may be insidious; hence, detailed guidelines for the diagnosis and follow-up are needed. Small, non-conclusive studies have been conducted on specific populations, such as immunodeficient, immunosuppressed or AIDS patients, as well as in patients with known lung infections and those with non-neoplastic diffuse lung disease. Significant results and the best clinical evidence on this matter were obtained by:

- The Brock model used with data from the Pan-Canadian Early Detection of Lung Cancer Study: this is the only multivariate analysis that includes multiple

pulmonary nodules and has shown a modest negative correlation between multiple nodules and probability of malignancy.
- The Nederlands-Leuvens Longkanker Screenings Onderzoek (NELSON) trial: it proposed the use of a diagnostic algorithm based on the morphology of the largest nodule.

On the other hand, in patients currently or previously suffering of cancer, multiple pulmonary nodules can more frequently be of secondary nature; based on their primary tumor, these nodules might present with different characteristics. In any case, also in this setting the diagnostic approach based on the patient's history and the position and morphology of nodules remains generally valid and allows to differentiate between the various types of primary pulmonary neoplasms with multifocal onset.

Suggested Readings

Callister ME, et al. How should pulmonary nodules be optimally investigated and managed? Lung Cancer. 2016;91:48–55. https://doi.org/10.1016/j.lungcan.2015.10.018.

MacMahon, Heber, et al. Guidelines for management of incidental pulmonary nodules detected on CT images: from the Fleischner Society 2017. Radiology. 2017;284(1):228–43.

Truong MT, et al. Update in the evaluation of the solitary pulmonary nodule. Radiographics. 2014;34(6):1658–79.

Lung Cancer

5

Andrea Porfiri, Carola Palla, Angelo Iannarelli,
and Hans-Peter Erasmus

Lung cancer is the most widespread neoplasm in the world and the first cause of cancer death for males; its incidence is globally increasing in the female population. The mortality rate is increasing in Asia and Africa and decreasing in Western countries, possibly due to the advancement of more precise and more readily available diagnostic tools and the development of new therapeutic strategies.

A complete surgical resection is associated with improved survival, but only about 25–60% of patients are eligible for intervention at the time of diagnosis. The most important prognostic factor in lung cancer is cancer stage at diagnosis. The TNM (Tumor, Nodes, Metastasis) system that evaluates the cancer's anatomical extension is the most widely used and internationally accepted tumor staging system. Since its first publication by Pierre Denoix in 1943, it has been constantly updated. In 2017, the International Association for the Study of Lung Cancer (IASLC) issued the 8th edition of the "TNM classification of malignant tumors," based on a larger sample size from several reference centers.

Traditionally, the TNM applied only to Non-Small Cell Lung Cancer (NSCLC) that accounts for 85% of lung cancer cases and would not be applicable to microcytomas or Small Cell Lung Cancer (SCLC). Indeed, for SCLC only "local" and "extended" disease are distinguished, often leaving systemic chemotherapy as the only viable option. However, since the 7th edition it can be used to evaluate SCLC as well.

Imaging plays a key role in the management of lung cancer and is highly reliable, thanks to the constant development of new diagnostic techniques, with PET and PET-CT being worth particular mention.

The clinical staging of neoplasms through imaging (cT, cN, cM) should not be confused with the definitive histological or pathological staging occurring after surgical resection or biopsy (pT, pN, pM). When surgically resected, a description of

A. Porfiri · C. Palla · A. Iannarelli · H.-P. Erasmus (✉)
Department of Radiological, Oncological and Pathological Sciences, Sapienza University of Rome, Rome, Italy

I. Carbone, M. Anzidei (eds.), *Thoracic Radiology*,
https://doi.org/10.1007/978-3-030-35765-8_5

the resection margins (R1: cancer cells present microscopically at the resection margin; R0: disease-free margins) should also be included. The correlation between clinical and pathological staging is around 35–55% and is expected to increase in the future. The current TNM is summarized in Tables 5.1, 5.2, and 5.3 (adapted from the 8th Edition Lung Cancer TNM Staging Summary) (Fig. 5.1).

Table 5.1 T staging, 8th TNM edition

T—primary tumor *(greatest diameter guides size assessment)*		
TX		Primary tumor cannot be assessed, or tumor proven by the presence of malignant cells in sputum or bronchial washings but not visualized by imaging or bronchoscopy
T0		No evidence of primary tumor
Tis		Carcinoma in situ
T1		≤3 cm Surrounded by lung or visceral pleura Without bronchoscopic evidence of invasion more proximal than the lobar bronchus (i.e., not in the main bronchus)
	T1mi	Minimally invasive (≤5 mm) adenocarcinoma
	T1a	≤1 cm
	T1b	Between 1 and 2 cm
	T1c	Between 2 and ≤3 cm
T2		>3 cm but ≤5 cm Or tumor with any of the following features: – Involves main bronchus regardless of distance to the carina, but without involving it – Invades visceral pleura – Associated with atelectasis or obstructive pneumonitis that extends to the hilar region, either in part or the entire lung
	T2a	>3 cm but ≤4 cm
	T2b	>4 cm but ≤5 cm
T3		>5 cm but ≤7 cm Or invading any of the following: – chest wall (including superior sulcus tumors) – phrenic nerve – parietal pericardium Or associated separate tumor nodule(s) in the same lobe as the primary
T4		>7 cm Or invading any of the following: – diaphragm – mediastinum – heart – great vessels – trachea – recurrent laryngeal nerve – esophagus – vertebral body – carina Separate tumor nodule(s) in a different ipsilateral lobe to that of the primary

Modified from: Goldstraw P, Chansky K, Crowley J, et al. The IASLC Lung Cancer Staging Project: proposals for the revision of the stage grouping in the forthcoming (8th) edition of the TNM classification of lung cancer. J Thorac Oncol. 2016;11:39–51, with permission from Elsevier

Table 5.2 N staging, 8th TNM edition

N—regional lymph nodes *(also counts when involvement by direct contact occurs)*		
NX		Regional lymph nodes not assessable
N0		No metastasis to regional lymph nodes
N1		Metastasis in following *ipsilateral* lymph nodes: – peribronchial – hilar – intrapulmonary
	N1a	Involvement of one N1 station nodes
	N1b	Involvement of multiple N1 stations nodes
N2		Metastasis in the following *ipsilateral* lymph nodes: – mediastinal – subcarinal
	N2a1	Involvement of a single N2 station nodes without N1 involvement
	N2a2	Involvement of a single N2 station nodes with N1 involvement
	N2b	Involvement of multiple N2 stations nodes
N3		Metastasis in the following *ipsilateral*: – scalene – supraclavicular OR following *contralateral* lymph nodes: – mediastinal – hilar – scalene – supraclavicular

Modified from: Goldstraw P, Chansky K, Crowley J, et al. The IASLC Lung Cancer Staging Project: proposals for the revision of the stage grouping in the forthcoming (8th) edition of the TNM classification of lung cancer. J Thorac Oncol. 2016;11:39–51, with permission from Elsevier

Table 5.3 M staging, 8th TNM edition

M—distant metastasis		
M0		No distant metastasis
M1		Distant metastasis
	M1a	Separate tumor nodule(s) in contralateral lobe Pleural or pericardial nodules Malignant pleural or pericardial effusion
	M1b	Single extrathoracic in single organ (or single non-regional lymph node)
	M1c	Multiple extrathoracic metastases in $\geq$1 organ

Modified from: Goldstraw P, Chansky K, Crowley J, et al. The IASLC Lung Cancer Staging Project: proposals for the revision of the stage grouping in the forthcoming (8th) edition of the TNM classification of lung cancer. J Thorac Oncol. 2016;11:39–51, with permission from Elsevier

Staging

Subsets of certain T, N, and M categories can be grouped into different stages of the disease, as these share similar treatment options and prognosis. In Table 5.4 and 5.5, we list a simplified and a more detailed version.

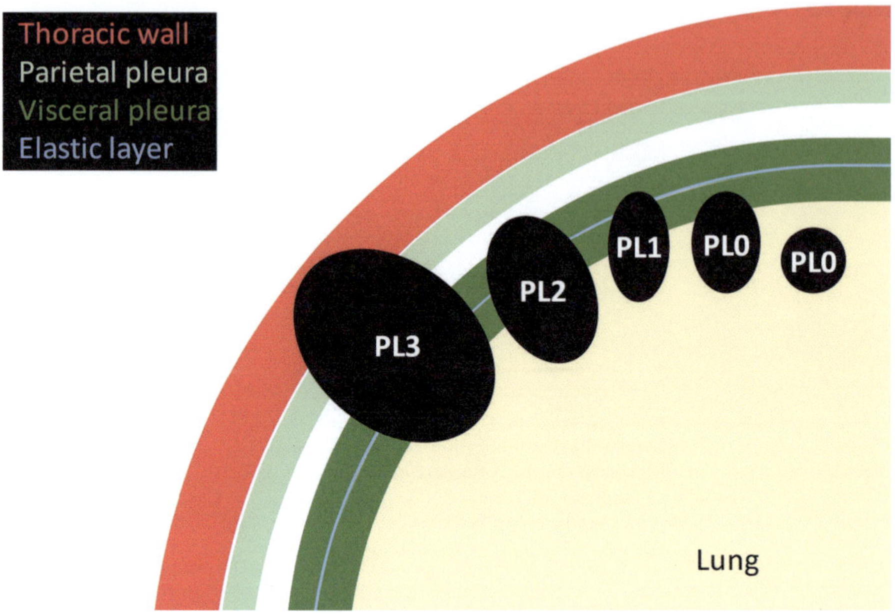

Fig. 5.1 *PL0*, tumor within the subpleural lung parenchyma OR invading superficially into the pleural connective tissue; *PL1*, tumor invades beyond the elastic layer; *PL2*, tumor invading the pleural pseudocavity; *PL3*, tumor invading any component of the parietal pleura. PL1 & PL2 = T2 and PL3 = T3

Table 5.4 Simplified TNM staging

	N0	N1	N2	N3
T1	IA	IIB	IIIA	IIIB
T2a	IB	IIB	IIIA	IIIB
T2b	IIA	IIB	IIIA	IIIB
T3	IIB	IIIA	IIIB	IIIC
T4	IIIA	IIIA	IIIB	IIIC
M1a	IVA	IVA	IVA	IVA
M1b	IVA	IVA	IVA	IVA
M1c	IVB	IVB	IVB	IVB

Modified from: Detterbeck, Frank C, et al. The eighth edition lung cancer stage classification. Chest. 2017;151.1:193–203, with permission from Elsevier

Table 5.5 Detailed TNM staging

Stage	T	N	M
Occult carcinoma	TX	N0	M0
0	Tis		
IA1	T1mi or T1a		
IA2	T1b		
IA3	T1c		
IB	T2a		
IIA	T2b		
IIB	Any T1 or T2	N1	
	T3	N0	
IIIA	Any T1 or T2	N2	
	T3 or T4	N1	
	T4	N0	
IIIB	Any T1 or T2	N3	
	T3 or T4	N2	
IIIC	T3 or T4	N3	
IVA	Any T	Any N	M1a or M1b
IVB	Any T	Any N	M1c

Modified from: Goldstraw P, Chansky K, Crowley J, et al. The IASLC Lung Cancer Staging Project: proposals for the revision of the stage grouping in the forthcoming (8th) edition of the TNM classification of lung cancer. J Thorac Oncol. 2016;11:39–51, with permission from Elsevier

Table 5.6 Lung adenocarcinoma classification IASLC/ATS/ERS 2011

Pre-invasive lesions: • Atypical adenomatous hyperplasia AAH (<5 mm) • Adenocarcinoma in situ AIS (<3 cm, no invasion)
Minimally invasive adenocarcinoma MIA (<3 cm, invasion <5 mm)
Invasive adenocarcinoma (>3 cm, invasion >5 mm)

Invasive Pulmonary Adenocarcinoma

Pulmonary adenocarcinoma is the most common variant among lung tumors, accounting for more than 50% of all histotypes. It belongs to the category of Non-Small Cell Lung Cancer (NSCLC), is found more frequently in women and non-smokers and develops predominantly in the lung periphery. A new classification for adenocarcinoma (IASLC/ATS/ERS, 2011, Table 5.6) has recently been proposed (and been confirmed in the latest TNM) and includes, in addition to invasive adenocarcinoma, pre-invasive forms such as atypical adenomatous hyperplasia, adenocarcinoma in situ (previously "bronchioalveolar carcinoma"), and minimally invasive adenocarcinoma.

In *Atypical Adenomatous Hyperplasia (AAH)*, atypical type II pneumocytes or Clara cells start proliferating locally along the alveolar wall and respiratory bronchioles. Radiologically, this usually appears as a small non-solid nodule (up to 5 mm) that can remain stable for years.

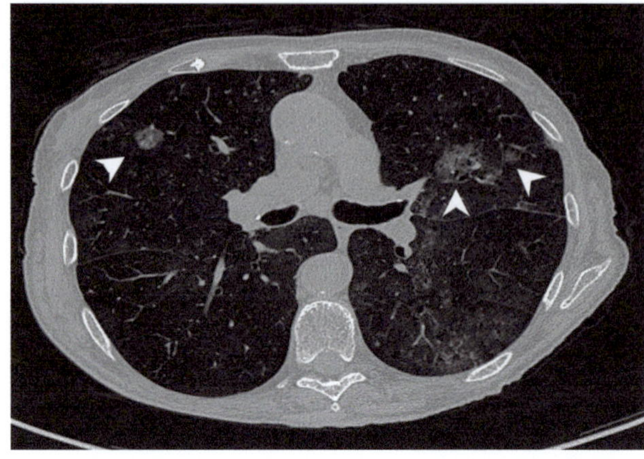

Fig. 5.2 Invasive pulmonary adenocarcinoma: multiple mixed parenchymal nodules (*arrowheads*)

In situ adenocarcinoma (ISA), existing as a mucinous or a non-mucinous variant, is formed by neoplastic cells that tend to spread along pre-existing anatomical structures, preserving an intact alveolar architecture without stromal or vascular invasion, a process known as lepidic growth. Radiologically, it appears as a localized, non-infiltrating lesion of up to 3 cm in size, generally non-solid and only rarely mixed.

Minimally invasive adenocarcinoma (MIA) has a predominantly lepidic growth, the overall size is <3 cm with an invasive component smaller than 5 mm. On CT scans, it appears mixed, prevalently non-solid with small solid elements (<5 mm).

Invasive adenocarcinoma includes several histologic patterns such as lepidic, acinar, papillary, micropapillary, and solid; however, the mixed variants are very common. Radiologically, it may occur as a single pulmonary nodule, a segmental or lobar parenchymal consolidation area, or predominantly interstitial diffuse lung disease. In the latter case, multiple more-or-less defined parenchymal solid or mixed nodules in a bronchocentric distribution pattern are the most frequent CT finding, and are often associated with a halo sign; multiple areas of parenchymal consolidation with air bronchograms is another possible presentation (Figs. 5.2 and 5.3).

Based solely on a CT scan, it can be very difficult to distinguish a primary pulmonary adenocarcinoma from diffuse alveolar metastases; in such cases, other key diagnostic criteria need to be evaluated, such as concurrent extrapulmonary tumors and/or mediastinal or thoracic lymphadenopathies located in sites that are not typical of primary pulmonary neoplasms.

Primary Syn- and Metachronous Lung Tumors

A non-negligible percentage (~8%) of newly diagnosed lung tumors arises in patients with a history of cancer, be it thoracic or extrathoracic.

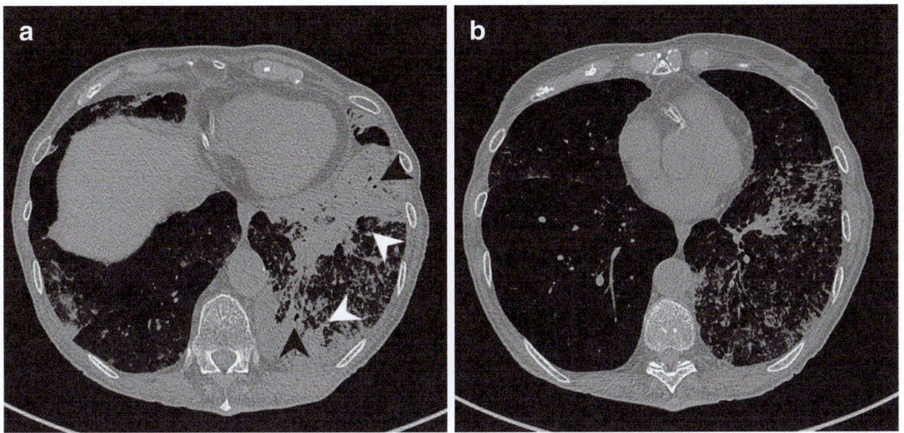

Fig. 5.3 Invasive pulmonary adenocarcinoma: (**a**) Parenchymal consolidations (*white arrowheads*) in a lobar/segmental distribution with air bronchograms (*black arrowheads*), (**b**) Diffuse interstitial involvement of the left lower lobe

Table 5.7 Martini and Melamed criteria for the definition of second primary lung cancer

Synchronous MPLC	Metachronous MPLC
A. Physically distinct and separate tumors	A. Histologically different
B. Histotype:	B. Histologically the same, if:
1. Different	1. Tumor-free interval between the neoplasms ≥2 years
2. Same but in different segment, lobe, or lung if: (a) Origin from carcinoma in situ (b) No evidence of carcinoma in common lymphatics (c) No extrapulmonary metastases at the time of diagnosis	2. Origin from carcinoma in situ 3. Second tumor in different lobe or lung but: (a) No evidence of carcinoma in common lymphatics (b) No extrapulmonary metastases at the time of diagnosis

Multiple Primary Lung Cancer (MPLC) cases are increasing in number, both because of improvements in diagnostic techniques and increased survival of oncologic patients.

Multiple primary lung tumors can be both synchronous and metachronous and because of their similar histologic characteristics it can be particularly difficult to distinguish them from metastases. This difficulty is further enhanced within areas of previous radiotherapy that alters tissue morphology.

The distinction between primary, synchronous, metachronous lung cancer, and intrapulmonary metastases is currently based on well-defined clinical and pathological criteria (Tables 5.7, 5.8, and 5.9).

New molecular and genomic analyses can aid in clearly differentiating between these; this is especially important for the correct choice of treatment that may be surgical as a first line in a second primary lung cancer.

Table 5.8 Modified criteria by Antakli et al. for the definition of second primary lung cancer

A. Different histological conditions
B. Same histological conditions with two or more of the following: 1. Anatomically distinct 2. Associated pre-malignant lesion 3. No systemic metastases 4. No mediastinal spread 5. Different DNA ploidy

Table 5.9 Modified criteria by Shen et al. for the definition of second primary lung cancer

A. Same histology, anatomically separated: 1. Cancers in different lobes 2. No N2, 3 involvement 3. No systemic metastases
B. Same histology, temporally separated: 1. Time interval between appearance of cancers ≥4 years 2. No systemic metastases from any tumor
C. Different histology: 1. Different histotype 2. Different molecular genetic characteristics 3. Arising separately from foci of carcinoma in situ

Lung Lymphoma

Lung lymphoma describes the involvement of the pulmonary parenchyma by a lymphoma. This can occur through two main mechanisms:

Secondary pulmonary lymphoma: the most common form, found in about 4% of patients with Non-Hodgkin Lymphoma (NHL). It is caused by hematogenous spread of the disease (both Hodgkin and Non-Hodgkin Lymphoma) or direct invasion of the pulmonary parenchyma from contiguous hilar or mediastinal lymph nodes. This disease is, thus, the progression of a known hematologic disorder arising from the mediastinum or other extrathoracic locations.

Primary pulmonary lymphoma: rarely encountered, it represents only 3–4% of extranodal lymphomas and 0.5–1% of all lung tumors. Lesions are found within the pulmonary parenchyma without extrapulmonary manifestations. Primary lung lymphomas include three main classes: low- and high-grade B-cell lung lymphoma and lymphomatoid granulomatosis.

Pulmonary lymphomas may appear as multiple bilateral, sometimes bronchocentric, nodules, diffuse opacities with a reticulonodular pattern, or parenchymal consolidation areas that may contain cavities or air bronchograms (Fig. 5.4). Pleural thickening and pleural effusion can be associated with such findings.

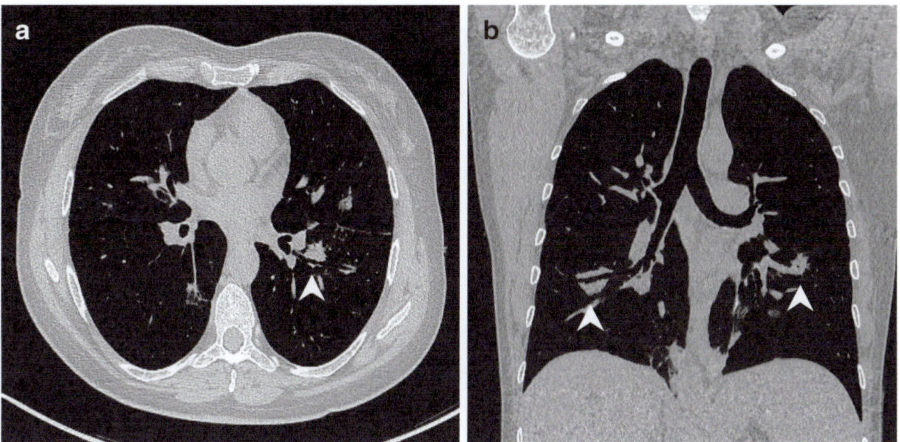

Fig. 5.4 Pulmonary lymphoma: bilateral parenchymal nodules, some of which bronchocentric (*arrowheads*)

Kaposi's Sarcoma

Kaposi's sarcoma is a mesenchymal tumor of medium to low aggressiveness that involves the vascular and lymphatic system. In about a third of Kaposi's sarcoma patients, there is lung involvement with nodular and interstitial pattern. On CT scans, ill-defined "flame-shaped" nodules are seen bilaterally. They are neither calcific, nor cavitary, often bronchocentric, and found in a symmetrical fashion in the parahilar and basal regions; surrounding semisolid irregular areas, thickening of the interlobular septa, pleural effusion, and lymphadenopathy may occur.

Metastases

A very high percentage (84–98%) of multiple lung lesions are metastatic in origin. Pulmonary metastases are very common and result from hematogenous or lymphatic dissemination from lung, breast, gastrointestinal, soft tissues, bone, and genitourinary neoplasms.

Hematogenous metastases are solid nodules, roughly rounded, of varying size, and more commonly found in the lung periphery. Peculiar characteristics can be related to specific primary cancer histotypes:

- Miliary: numerous tiny nodules spread over the entire lung fields are more common in melanoma, medullary thyroid cancer, and renal cancer (Fig. 5.5).
- Large (up to more than 10 cm): typical of sarcoma, colorectal and renal cancer, and melanoma (Fig. 5.6).
- Cavitated: more common in squamous cell carcinoma of the head and neck, cervix and bladder, gastric adenocarcinoma, and sarcoma (Fig. 5.7).

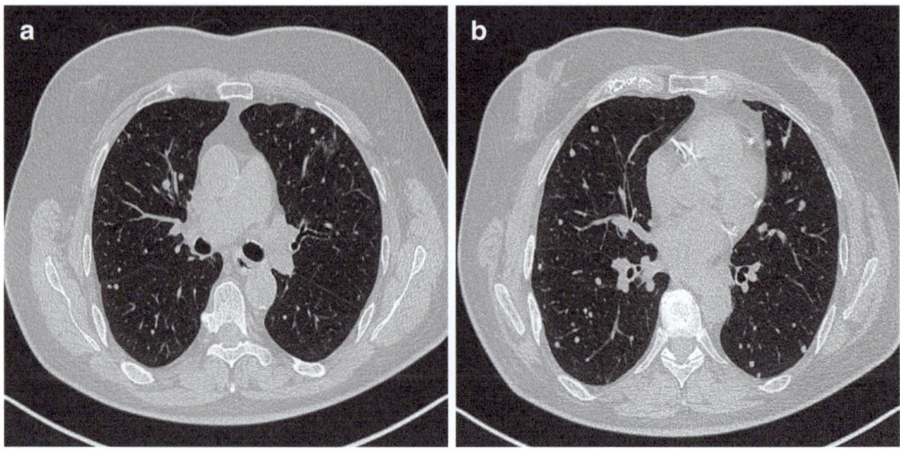

Fig. 5.5 Metastases secondary to medullary thyroid cancer

Fig. 5.6 Metastases secondary to sarcoma

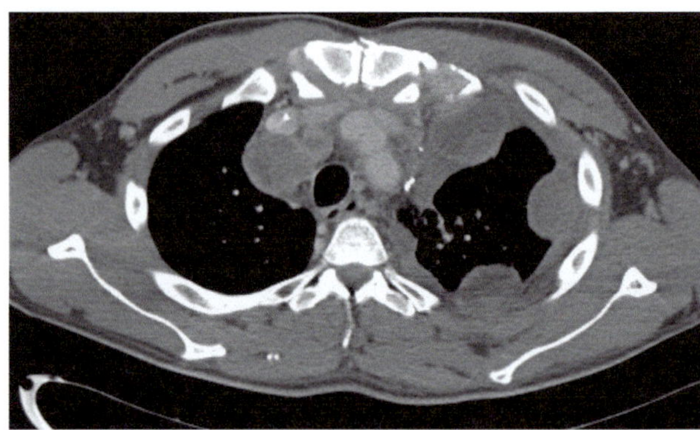

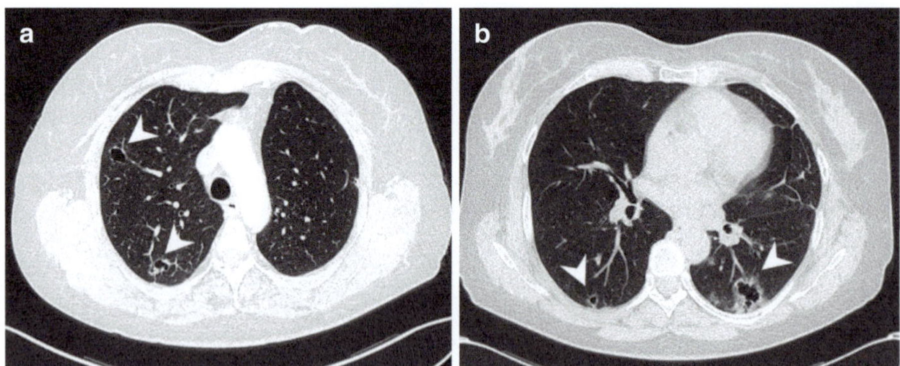

Fig. 5.7 Cavitated metastases secondary to cervical cancer (*arrowheads*)

- Calcific: typical of osteosarcoma, chondrosarcoma, papillary thyroid cancer and mucinous cancers of the gastrointestinal tract, breast, and ovaries; intranodular calcifications may be the result of chemotherapy (Fig. 5.8).
- Lepidic growth: uncommon, can be attributed to the spread of pulmonary adenocarcinoma and gastrointestinal adenocarcinomas. They present as areas of consolidation resembling pneumonia, sometimes with air bronchograms; they can also appear as semisolid nodules with a peripheral halo.
- Hemorrhagic: with peripheral "halo sign," most commonly found in highly vascularized tumors, such as choriocarcinomas, angiosarcomas, and melanomas (Fig. 5.9).

Lymphogenous metastases present with a diffuse interstitial infiltration with reticulonodular pattern, as seen in carcinomatous lymphangitis. A micronodular, irregular thickening of both the interlobular septa and peribronchovascular interstitium occurs and is sometimes associated with pleural carcinomatosis and spread

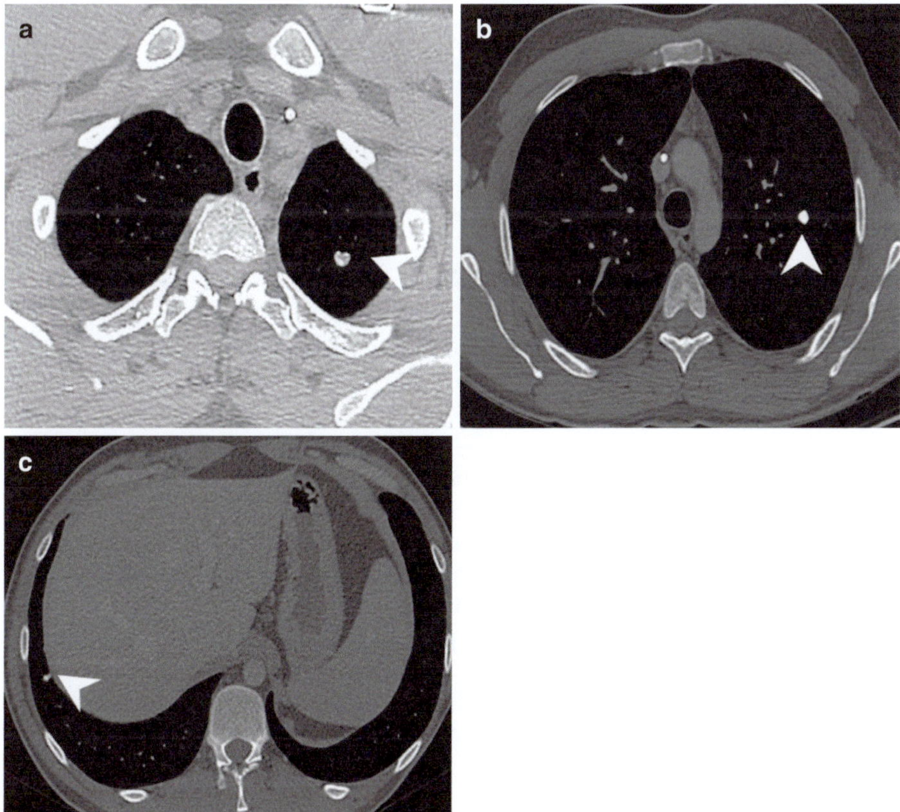

Fig. 5.8 Calcified metastases secondary to mucinous tumor (*arrowheads*)

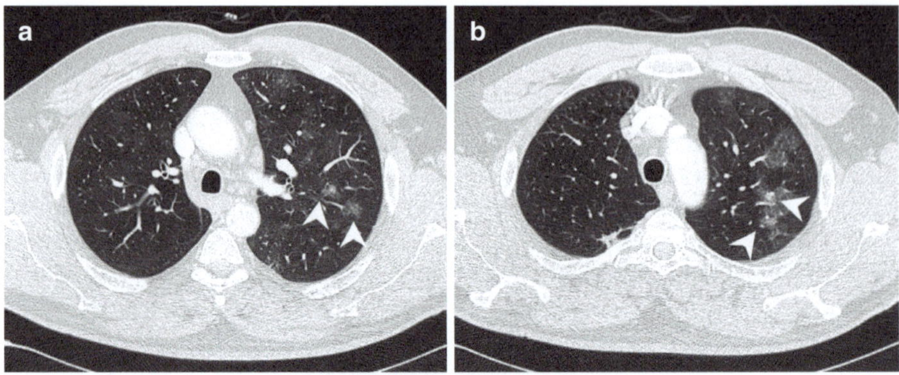

Fig. 5.9 Hemorrhagic metastases secondary to melanoma (*arrowheads*)

Fig. 5.10 Carcinomatous lymphangitis secondary to breast cancer

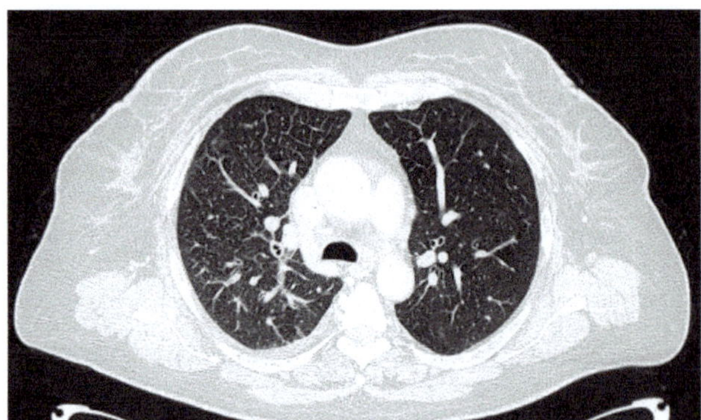

along the fissures. This is most commonly observed in adenocarcinomas of the stomach, breast, and pancreas (Fig. 5.10).

Resectable and Unresectable Disease

Evaluating the resectability of a lung cancer is a complex analytical process; the criteria to be used are still heavily debated. Imaging has a central role and only rarely histology is necessary to evaluate the extent of disease.

The new TNM may be helpful in both prognostic stratification and evaluating the resectability of a lung cancer. In general, stages I and II are always resectable while stage IV is by definition inoperable (Table 5.10). Stages IIIA and IIIB describe a "locally advanced" disease without distant metastases. In these cases, an evaluation of the patient's individual characteristics is necessary to decide the best therapeutic strategy.

Table 5.10 Stage and resectability

Stage	Resectable?
Ia	Yes
Ib	
IIa	
IIb	
IIIa	Selected patients
IIIb	No
IV	

Types of Resection

Surgery is planned based on the tumor characteristics and patient compliance.

Minimal resections such as **segmentectomy** or **wedge resection** are an option for stage I lung cancer. While wedge resection provides better postoperative compliance with a lower incidence of respiratory failure in patients with reduced pulmonary function, segmentectomy shows better results in terms of lower locoregional recurrence rates. These improved outcomes may be due to a complete removal of the lymphatic vessels that drain the tumor, not performed during wedge resections.

Most lung tumors are treated with **lobectomy**, which results in better oncological outcomes than the previously listed methods; when not sufficient for complete eradication of the neoplasm, **pneumonectomy** is performed.

Pneumonectomy is generally indicated when neoplastic tissue infiltrates the major or minor fissure, resulting in involvement of both upper and lower lobes. In addition, the infiltration of hilar structures, such as the main pulmonary artery, upper and lower pulmonary veins, and/or the main bronchus, makes a pneumonectomy mandatory. A special exception is the infiltration of the main bronchus only; here, a lobectomy can be performed after a sleeve resection with bronchoplasty. Likewise, a focal involvement of the main pulmonary artery can be treated with resection and angioplasty. Before pneumonectomies, an evaluation of the patient's fitness for surgery is needed, especially in cases of heart failure and low pulmonary reserve.

Resectability Considering the Extension of the Primitive Tumor

Mediastinal Involvement

Despite being T4 (stage III, locally advanced disease), a focal involvement of the mediastinal pleura and/or fat does not preclude surgical resection. However, whenever the removal of a large proportion of mediastinal fatty tissue is to be expected, this should be considered as a condition of non-resectability because of the high rate of locoregional recurrence.

On CT scans, mediastinal involvement is defined as:

- contact margins of >3 cm between tumor and mediastinum
- tumor extends into mediastinal adipose tissue
- pericardial and pleural thickening

Unfortunately, CT scans has low accuracy in diagnosing minimal mediastinal infiltrations. When this is suspected, inducing a pneumothorax and scanning at maximum inhalation and exhalation have been reported to increase sensitivity. Infiltration of vital structures (heart, great vessels, esophagus, vertebrae, or trachea) is generally a contraindication to surgery. Imaging criteria for infiltration are contact around >90° of the aorta, no adipose tissue between tumor and mediastinal structures, presence of mass effect. Some authors reported that CT and MRI scans are equally valid in evaluating mediastinal infiltration; however, both methods offer low accuracy since infiltration and contiguity are often being hard to distinguish.

There are some exceptions in case of infiltration of vital structures where surgery can still be a therapeutic option: when the carina is infiltrated, it is sometimes possible to resect the distal 3–4 cm of the trachea with pneumonectomy and sleeve resection with bronchoplasty (with termino-terminal anastomosis between the contralateral main bronchus and the trachea). Furthermore, a small portion of the left atrium can be resected if infiltrated. If the disease extends to the intrapericardial segment of the pulmonary arteries, it can be resectable if the portions not involved are long enough for clamping (Fig. 5.15). When only the tunica adventitia of the aorta is involved, it is possible to perform an accurate adventitial dissection. The infiltration of the upper vena cava can be treated by using grafts. Finally, a focal infiltration of a vertebral body can be removed "en-bloc."

Chest Wall Involvement

Stoelben and Ludwig have shown that the invasion of the chest wall is rare, affecting 5% of patients that underwent resection of lung cancer; in T3N0M0 patients treated with surgery the survival is good, even when the tumor size was above 7 cm (T4 according to 8th TNM, which the study predates). Therefore, the invasion of the chest wall generally does not preclude resection.

Several authors have demonstrated a marked improvement in survival when patients with invasion of the thoracic wall underwent surgery with negative resection margins, even when N2. On CT scans, the only certain criterion for diagnosing chest wall infiltration is the direct visualization of extension outside of the rib cage, with or without rib or vertebral erosion. Inducing a pneumothorax can help visualizing a parietal invasion, similarly to mediastinal invasions. With Pancoast's tumors, MRI has better sensitivity than CT in evaluating surrounding structures. When an infiltration of the upper fissure is suspected, many consider radio- and chemotherapy before submitting the patient to surgery.

Infiltration of the Diaphragm

Patients with diaphragm infiltration, in good general health and no lymph node involvement, should be resectable with "en bloc" removal of the diaphragm, as suggested by many authors.

Rocco et al. have reported that in cases of diaphragmatic infiltration removal with wide resection margins, followed by the placement of a diaphragmatic artificial prosthesis, can be an excellent strategy; the authors reported a five-year survival of 20%.

Resection Considering Lymph Node Involvement

Patients with ipsilateral mediastinal metastases (N2) are considered resectable with the exception of a "bulky" involvement. However, there is no clear definition of "bulky" disease. In the literature, the most frequently used expressions are: dominant lymph node with a short axis >25 mm (according to other authors >30 mm); lymph nodes with extracapsular extension of neoplastic tissue; two or more N2 lymph nodes involved (Fig. 5.11).

Patients with "bulky" N2 nodal disease undergo neoadjuvant chemotherapy and only if the lymph node masses regress properly can surgery be considered; otherwise, the treatment of choice will be radiotherapy.

Patients with contralateral mediastinal and hilar, scalene or supraclavicular lymphadenopathies (N3) are placed in stage IIIB and are therefore considered inoperable (Figs. 5.12, 5.13, 5.14, 5.15, and 5.16).

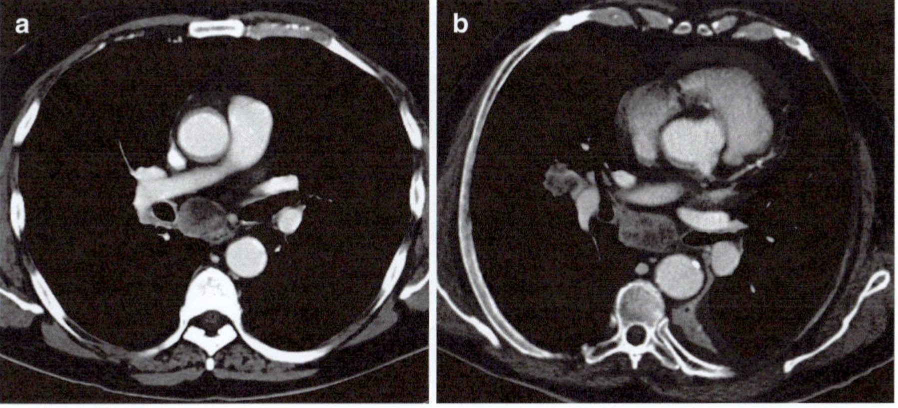

Fig. 5.11 "Bulky" N2: (**a**) Subcarinal lymph node >25 mm. (**b**) Subcarinal and ipsilateral hilar lymph node >25 mm

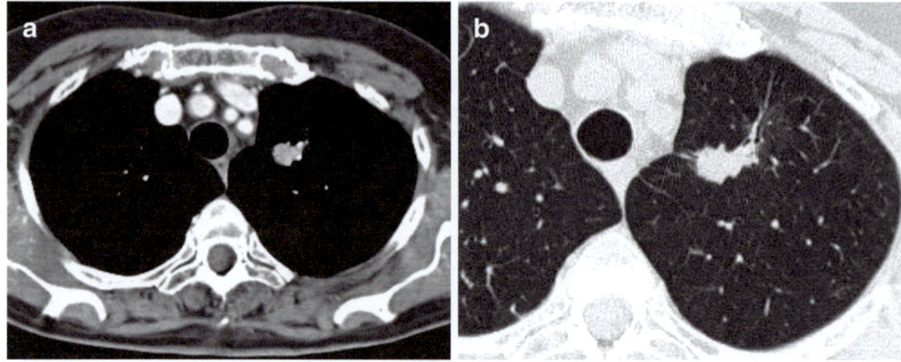

Fig. 5.12 T1b: T 2–3 cm

Fig. 5.13 T3: satellite nodule in the same lobe (*arrow*) as the primary tumor (*arrowhead*)

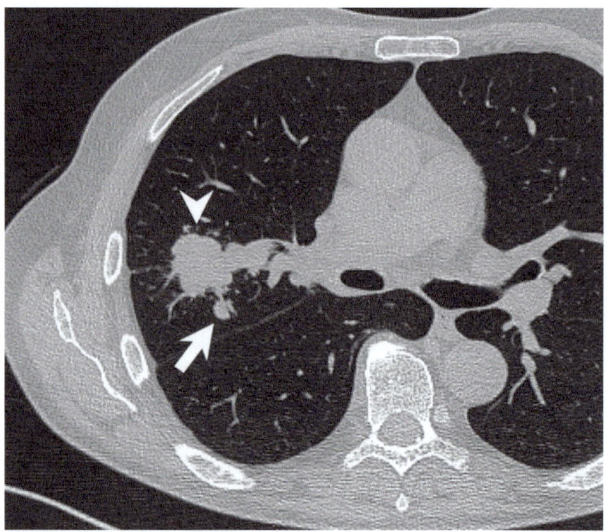

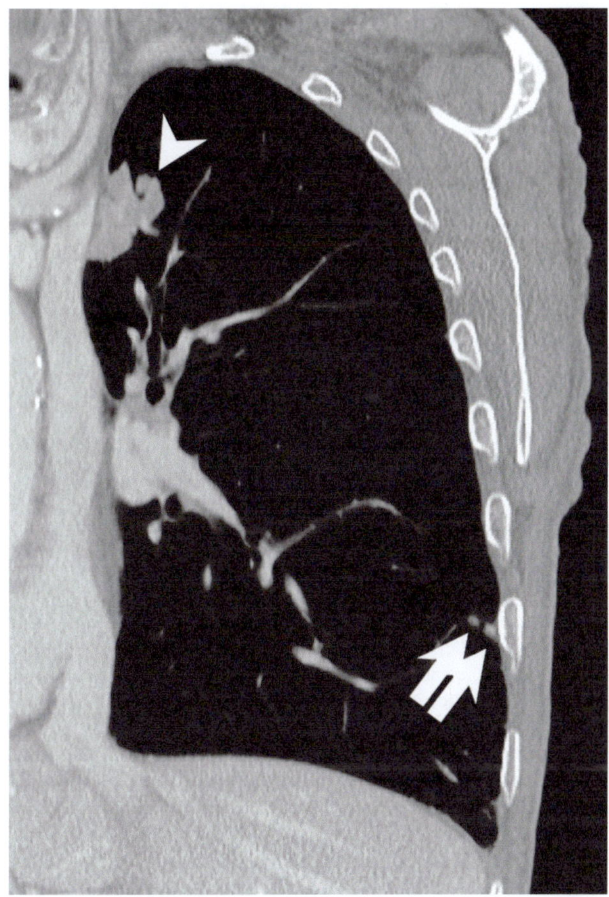

Fig. 5.14 T4: ipsilateral satellite nodules in a different lobe (*arrows*) as the primary tumor (*arrowhead*)

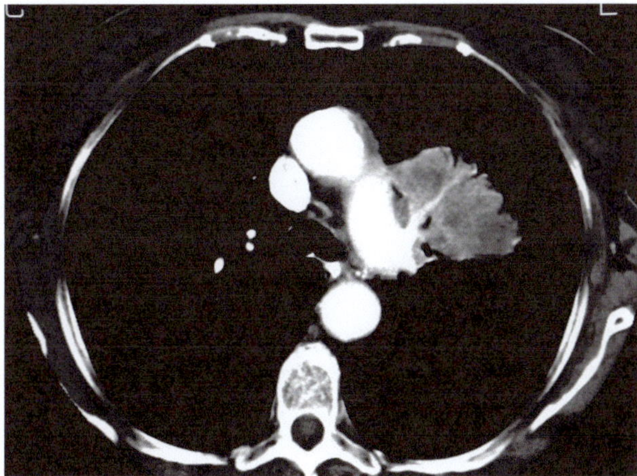

Fig. 5.15 T4: pulmonary artery infiltration

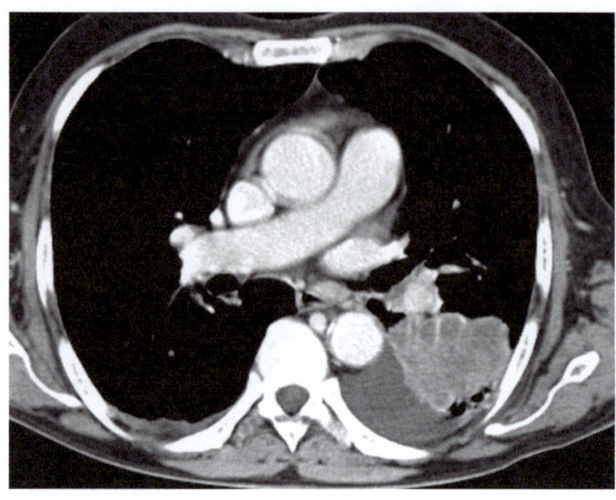

Fig. 5.16 M1a: neoplastic effusion

Suggested Readings

Lim W, et al. The 8th lung cancer TNM classification and clinical staging system: review of the changes and clinical implications. Quant Imaging Med Surg. 2018;8(7):709–18.

Robinson LA, et al. Treatment of non-small cell lung cancer-stage IIIA: ACCP evidence-based clinical practice guidelines (2nd edition). Chest. 2007;132(3 Suppl):243S.

Rusch VW, et al. The IASLC Lung Cancer Staging Project: a proposal for a new international lymph node map in the forthcoming 7th edition of the TNM classification for lung cancer. J Thorac Oncol. 2009;4(5):568.

Quint LE. Lung cancer: assessing resectability. Cancer Imaging. 2003;4:15–8.

Zugazagoitia J, et al. The new IASLC/ATS/ERS lung adenocarcinoma classification from a clinical perspective: current concepts and future prospects. J Thorac Dis. 2014;6(Suppl 5):S526–36.

Mediastinal Masses

6

Andrea Fiorelli and Giovanni Barchetti

The radiologic evaluation of mediastinal masses is complex and requires a thorough knowledge of the anatomy and compartments of the mediastinum.

Although in most cases the diagnosis of mediastinal masses is incidental, especially in the anterior mediastinum, whenever a clinical suspicion exists a standard CXR still remains the first imaging modality used. It allows to evaluate any deformation of the mediastinal profile and displacement of the normal anatomical structures. In some cases, a chest X-ray permits to characterize the location and type of mediastinal lesions; however a CT scan is deemed necessary for significant radiographic alterations.

Indications for CT Scan

A CT scan is indicated to confirm and characterize neoplastic and non-neoplastic mediastinal lesions identified on CXR. Specifically, it allows to correctly define their location, anatomical boundaries, tissue characteristics (cystic, vascularized, calcified, or fatty), and the presence of associated findings useful for diagnosis. Sometimes, a CT scan might not provide a definitive preoperative diagnosis; however, it helps to set the therapeutic management of the patient by indicating the next diagnostic procedure (PET, biopsy, mediastinoscopy, surgery). In patients with symptoms suggesting a mediastinal lesion but with a negative CXR, a CT scan might be prescribed based solely on the clinical presentation (i.e., suspect of thymoma in myasthenia gravis).

A. Fiorelli (✉) · G. Barchetti
Department of Radiological, Oncological and Pathological Sciences, Sapienza University of Rome, Rome, Italy

I. Carbone, M. Anzidei (eds.), *Thoracic Radiology*,
https://doi.org/10.1007/978-3-030-35765-8_6

Indications for MRI

MRI has a better tissue characterization and higher contrast resolution compared to CT scans and therefore is the most suitable imaging modality for mediastinal lesions not easily evaluable by CT for their tissue characteristics or their anatomical location. Indeed, MRI is advised for lesions with mixed content or rising from structures of the posterior mediastinum (esophagus, mediastinal and spinal nerves, vertebrae), from the heart (cardiac tumors, pericarditis), and from great vessels (vasculitis). Other indications for MRI are contraindications to iodinated contrast media and whenever one needs to avoid radiation exposure, such as in pediatric patients.

Mediastinal Diseases

Mediastinal diseases can be diagnosed using a classification scheme referring to the anatomical compartments of origin (Table 6.1):

- The **anterior mediastinum** is often indicated as the "*four T space,*" as it is the main site of **T**eratomas, lymphomas (**T**errible lymphoma), and diseases affecting the **T**hyroid gland and **T**hymus.
- The **middle mediastinum** is the main site of heart and great vessels pathologies.
- The **posterior mediastinum** is the main site of diseases involving the esophagus, vertebral column, and nervous structures.

The mediastinum can be secondarily affected by the complications of extra-mediastinal diseases of the chest wall, neck, and abdomen; in particular,

Table 6.1 Anatomical classification of mediastinal lesions, in relation to their content (fluid, fatty) and to their vascular origin

Mediastinal compartment	Type of lesion	Fluid content	Fatty content	Vascular origin
Anterior	**T**hymoma (**T**errible) lymphoma **T**eratoma **T**hyroid goiter	Cystic thymoma Cystic lymphoma Pericardial cyst	Teratoma Thymolipoma	Ascending aorta
Middle	Lymph nodes Duplication cyst Ascending aorta	Necrotic lymph nodes Duplication cyst Pericardial recess	Esophageal lipoma Lipomatosis	Aortic arch Azygos vein Heart
Posterior	Neurogenic tumors Bone	Schwannoma Meningocele	Extramedullary hematopoiesis	Ascending Aorta

uncontrolled inflammatory processes can extend to the mediastinum and cause mediastinitis and pneumomediastinum.

Thymoma

Thymomas are the most common primitive tumor of the anterior mediastinum. They are commonly encountered in patients older than 20 years of age with no gender predominance; around half of the patients are asymptomatic. In 40% of cases, thymoma is associated with paraneoplastic syndromes, including myasthenia gravis (30%), pure red cell aplasia (5%), and hypogammaglobulinemia (5–10%).

The dimension of the thymus varies according to the age; hence, it is fundamental to distinguish a physiologic residue or a juvenile thymus from a small mass; this is particularly difficult among pediatric patients and young adults. In the differential diagnoses, it is important to include the rebound thymic hyperplasia following chemotherapy (10%) which might mimic a mass in the anterior mediastinum. On CXRs, the thymoma can present as a slowly growing, oval-shaped opacity in the anterior mediastinum that may simulate cardiomegaly. The lateral projection can help to determine if the mass is a true thymoma since the tumor mass often causes a reduction or an obliteration of the retrosternal space (Fig. 6.1).

On CT images, the benign thymoma appears as a homogeneous mass, oval or lobulated, with regular margins; a peripheral capsule might be visible, and in 25% of cases there are punctate calcifications. The calcifications can be peripheral and eggshell-shaped in invasive lesions (Fig. 6.2).

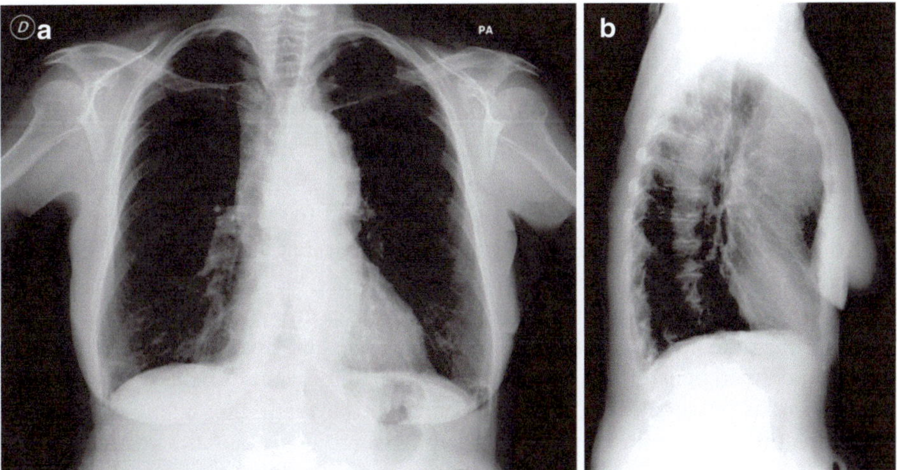

Fig. 6.1 Chest X-ray (standard projections): (**a**) PA view, an enlargement of the left mediastinal profile can be appreciated, (**b**) LL view, an obliteration of the retrosternal space is observed

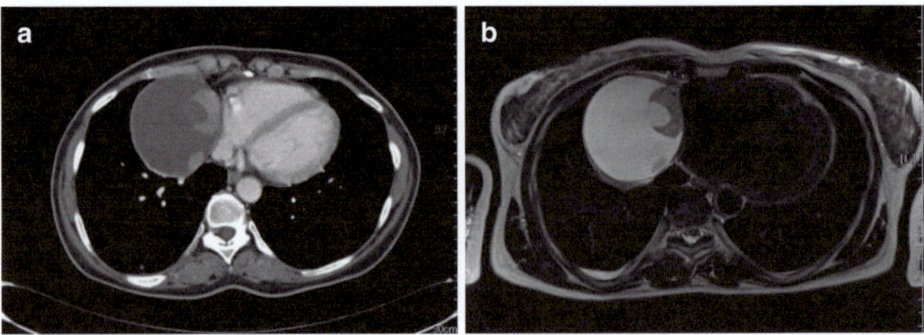

Fig. 6.2 Example of cystic thymoma in CT scan (**a**) and MRI (**b**): a cystic lesion located in the right cardiophrenic space with associated vascularized solid tissue

Before the administration of contrast medium, the thymoma has an attenuation of 45–75 HU (similar to the muscular tissue of the thoracic wall) and after contrast administration has a mild and homogenous enhancement. When invasive, it has a heterogeneous enhancement due to necrotic areas.

Other pathologies affecting the thymus are cysts, representing around 1% of mediastinal masses. The most common types are congenital, unilocular or secondary to the presence of a persistent thymopharyngeal duct. The acquired thymic cysts are usually multilocular, following inflammatory processes.

The thymus can be affected by lymphoproliferative disorders primarily or secondarily, with enlargement of both lobes or cystic lesions that might result difficult to discriminate from thymoma.

Lymphoma

Lymphadenopathies are the most common cause of anterior mediastinal masses and can be associated with lymphoproliferative disorders, such as Hodgkin Lymphoma (HL) and Non-Hodgkin Lymphoma (NHL), sarcoidosis and other inflammatory conditions, infections, and metastases. The lymphadenopathies of the anterior mediastinum are most commonly found in HL, mainly in the nodular sclerosis HL (around 70%) (Fig. 6.3). As the lymphomatous masses are frequently composed by multiple combined lymphadenopathies, they present lobular or polycyclic contours: this appearance can help to differentiate the pathologic lymph nodes from other mediastinal masses. Normally, the lymphomatous masses are homogeneous in density but, when they reach a significant dimension, they might show necrosis (lower attenuation areas) or hemorrhages (higher attenuation areas). Some features of lymphomas might resemble sarcoidosis, as both conditions can cause mediastinal lymphadenopathies; however, compared to lymphomas, sarcoidosis presents with lymph nodes in the anterior mediastinum only rarely, is seldom associated with pleural effusion and mainly involves more distally located bronchial lymph nodes.

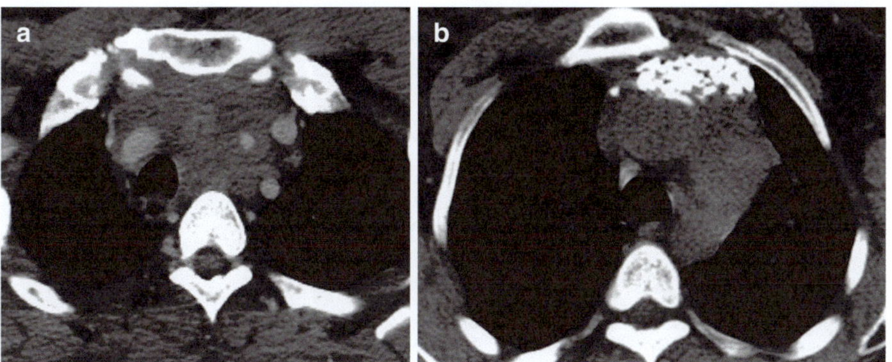

Fig. 6.3 Example of Hodgkin's lymphoma in the anterior mediastinum on axial CT scan: the tissue appears homogenous and encircles the vascular structures (**a**). After therapy (**b**), diffuse calcifications may be present

Germ Cell Tumors

Germ cell tumors commonly arise between the second and fourth decade, with a high prevalence of benign disease among females and malignant disease among males. Usually, these neoplasms originate in the anterior mediastinum, and then extend to the middle and posterior mediastinum, especially if malignant.

On CT scans, they present as roundish and lobulated masses. If benign, they show low attenuation and homogeneous density; if malignant, they might present calcifications with necrotic, cystic, or hemorrhagic areas.

The obliteration of the adipose cleavage planes that separate the mediastinal vascular structures can be indicative of malignancy although it may also be present in benign conditions due to fibrous adherences between the mass and vascular structures. For these reasons, CT scans are not able to accurately distinguish a malignant mass from a benign one. The most common germ cell tumors of the anterior mediastinum are teratomas, seminomas, and non-seminomatous tumors.

Teratoma

Teratoma represents 60% of germ cell tumors and is often an incidental finding in asymptomatic patients. It can be mature (solid), cystic (dermoid cyst), immature, malignant (teratocarcinoma), and mixed. Around 75% of teratomas are mature and are more common in females; the malignant form is more common among males. These lesions are considered of mediastinal origin as far as no lesions are presents in the gonads or the retroperitoneum. A CT scan is generally able to identify and characterize their origin although it may not be able to predict their malignancy, thus requiring markers and histologic data for correct diagnosis. The role of imaging is central for the evaluation of the treatment response and to identify recurrences (Fig. 6.4).

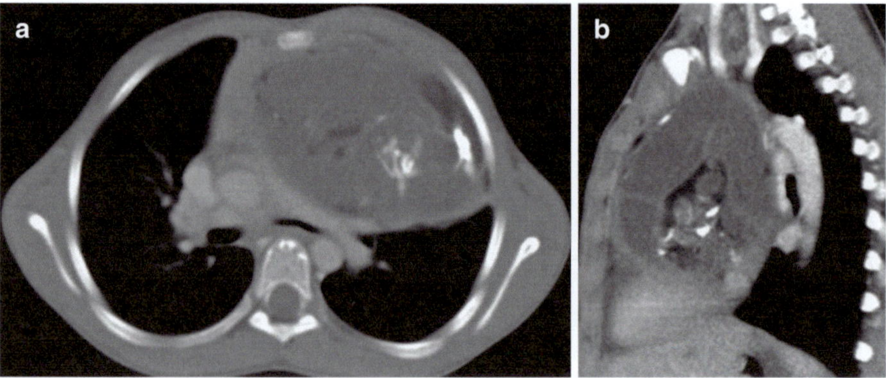

Fig. 6.4 CT (**a** axial; **b** sagittal) scan showing a germ cell tumor (mature solid teratoma) located in the anterior mediastinum. The lesion appears inhomogeneous with various tissues present (cartilage, bone, fat, and glandular tissue)

Seminoma

Seminoma represents 20% of germ cell tumors and is a disease exclusive to males, most frequently in the third decade of life. Often, the clinical onset is with thoracic pain and dyspnea; on imaging, it presents as a voluminous lesion located in the anterior mediastinum with a homogenous structure and regular margins. Metastases to bones, lung and thoracic lymph nodes are more common, calcifications and the invasion of the thoracic wall are rare.

Non-seminomatous Tumors

They represent 10% of germ cell tumors and occur more frequently between the third and fourth decade of life in male patients, with respiratory symptoms at onset. They can be associated with hematologic neoplasms and Klinefelter syndrome. A non-seminomatous tumor presents as a voluminous lesion located in the anterior mediastinum, with poorly defined margins. In more than 50% of cases, the lesion shows a necrotic central area and can obliterate the surrounding adipose planes, with associated pleural/pericardial effusion and lung metastases.

Thyroid Diseases

Cervicomediastinal goiters represent 10% of mediastinal masses, extending to the anterior mediastinum in most cases and to the posterior compartment only rarely. Most patients are asymptomatic, whereas a small percentage may have symptoms secondary to tracheal compression such as dyspnea, wheezing, and respiratory stridor. On CXR, the lesion presents as an anterosuperior or posterosuperior

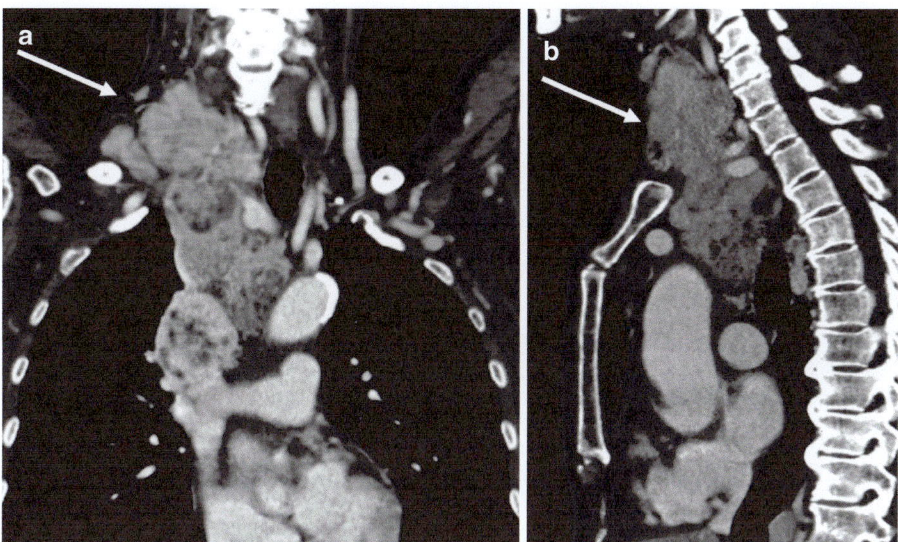

Fig. 6.5 CT scan (**a**, coronal; **b**, sagittal) of papillary thyroid neoplasia (*arrow*) at an advanced stage with involvement of the anterosuperior mediastinum, pathological laterocervical lymphadenopathies, and tracheal infiltration

mediastinal mass with possible associated lateral tracheal deviation at the thoracic inlet. Frequently, they are benign goiters or adenomas that appear on CT scan as masses in continuity with the thyroid gland with multinodular aspect, calcifications, (coarse, focal, annular) and small colloidal degeneration areas.

Malignant thyroid neoplasms, instead, extend to the mediastinum only rarely, and in such cases there is generally a voluminous mass in the superior and anterior mediastinum with possible direct invasion of the surrounding structures (larynx, esophagus, trachea). Metastases to the lymph nodes of the neck and mediastinum are particularly frequent, mainly in papillary and medullary carcinomas (up to 50%) (Fig. 6.5).

Pericardial Cyst

Pericardial cysts are more frequently secondary to an embryogenic defect of the coelomic cavity but can also follow inflammatory episodes involving the pericardium. They are located in the right cardiophrenic angle and are prevalent among adults between 30 and 40 years of age, almost always asymptomatic; only a small percentage of cases develops symptoms due to compression of the adjacent structures. On CT scan, they appear as a well-defined unilocular mass with fluid content. They can be oval, round, or triangular in shape, and the diameter can extend up to 30 cm (Fig. 6.6).

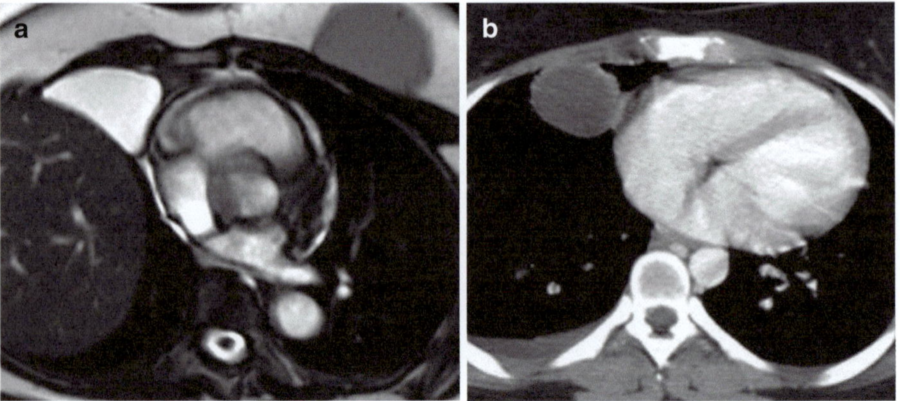

Fig. 6.6 Example of pericardial cyst located in the right cardiophrenic space. (**a**) The MR image shows a lesion with fluid content, (**b**) On contrast-enhanced CT scan, there is no significant parietal enhancement

Fibrosing Mediastinitis

Fibrosing mediastinitis is a diffuse fibrotic infiltration of the anterior, middle, or posterior mediastinum with a peak incidence between the second and fifth decade. Symptoms include cough, dyspnea, hemoptysis, and dysphagia. The etiology is usually infective (histoplasmosis, nocardiosis, tuberculosis), but it can be autoimmune or secondary to lymphatic obstruction. A CT scan shows mediastinal infiltration of fibrous tissue, surrounding and often compressing the great vessels, such as the superior vena cava; hilar masses can be present with an attenuation similar to the infiltrating tissue, sometimes with dense calcifications. Trachea and bronchi can be compromised with subsequent atelectasis and pneumonia.

Inflammatory Conditions

Abscess

Usually, it is a possible complication of sternotomy and involves the anterior mediastinum. Often the patients develop sepsis, which has a high mortality rate (up to 70%).

Tuberculosis

Tuberculous mediastinal lymphadenopathy commonly develops among pediatric patients and in patients with acquired immunodeficiencies. The lymphadenopathies show a central hypodense area, corresponding to necrosis, and are usually located at

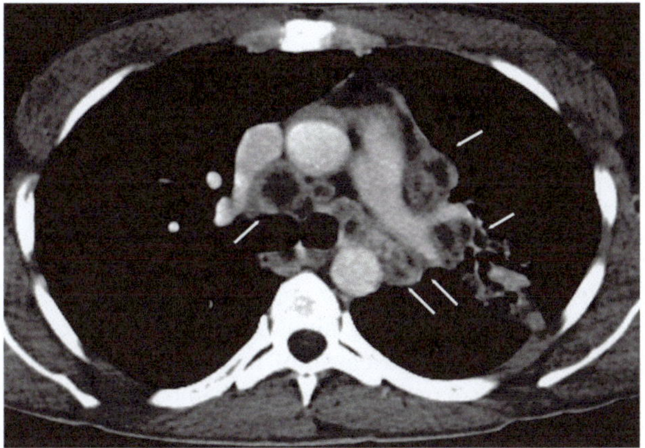

Fig. 6.7 Example of tuberculous mediastinal lymphadenopathies (*arrows*): it is possible to identify a central hypodense area that corresponds to the necrotic component

the right paratracheal site, the anterior mediastinum or hilum (Fig. 6.7). After the acute phase, the lymph nodes tend to calcify.

Sarcoidosis

Up to 80–90% of affected patients have thoracic lymphadenopathies. CT scans usually show enlarged lymph nodes with well-defined margins in the paratracheal and bilateral hilar zones. Calcifications are rare and occur only in chronic cases, in which they are eggshell shaped.

Metastases

Bronchogenic carcinoma is the first cause of metastatic mediastinal lymphadenopathies. Other extrathoracic tumors that can metastasize to the mediastinum are breast cancer, renal cancer, melanoma, and head and neck tumors. CT scans do not allow a precise characterization of the lymphadenopathies, but three criteria can help to identify a suspicious lymph node as metastatic:

- **Dimension**: >9 mm diameter measured on the short axis of the lymph node. However, this criterion does not consider that there are metastatic lymph nodes of small dimensions, mainly in their initial stages, and inflammatory lymph nodes of great dimensions.
- **Morphology**: generally, an inflammatory lymph node is oval in shape with a clear difference in the lengths of its diameters, whereas a metastatic lymph node is round with equivalent diameters.
- **Density**: necrosis is associated more often with metastatic lymphadenopathies, especially if large in dimensions; however, also some inflammatory disorders, as tuberculosis, are frequently associated with necrotic lymphadenopathies.

Vascular Disorders

The most common vascular disorders in the mediastinum affect the great vessels, in particular the thoracic aorta, and include aneurysms, intramural hematomas, and dissections. These pathologies are discussed in Chap. 11.

Hematoma

Venous lesions following blunt trauma or, less frequently, direct iatrogenic lesions are the most common cause of mediastinal hematomas. Spontaneous hematomas can also occur in patients receiving hemodialysis. On CT, a hematoma presents as a fluid collection hyperdense at baseline, with possibly associated air bubbles. Edema of the thoracic wall soft tissues and sternal or rib fractures can be associated findings. In most cases, after contrast administration it is possible to identify and localize the origin of the bleeding.

Esophageal Diseases

Esophageal Cancer

Esophageal cancer can appear as an intraluminal mass or as a thickening of the esophageal wall with or without stenosis of the lumen. A CT scan is useful to stage the thoracic esophageal cancer and assess the thickness and the longitudinal extension of the pathological tissue and the involvement of the periesophageal tissues, lymph nodes, and tracheobronchial tree (Fig. 6.8).

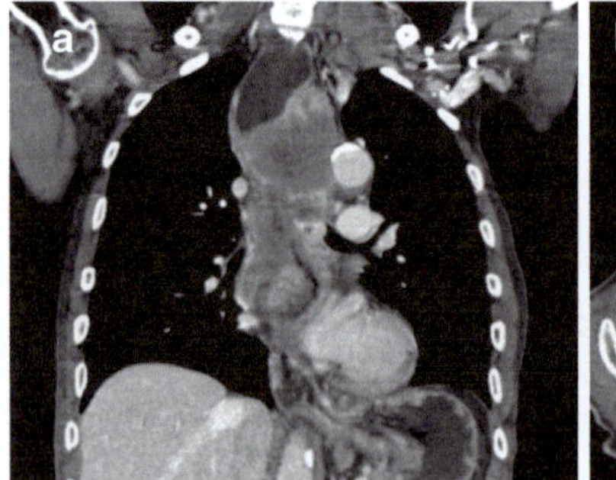

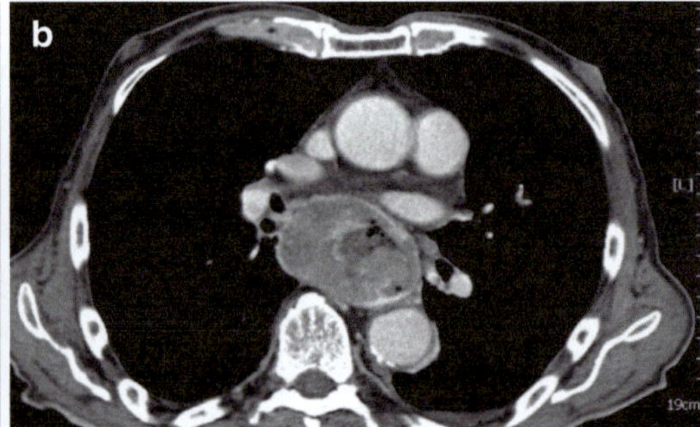

Fig. 6.8 Example of esophageal cancer in CT scan (**a**, coronal; **b**, axial): esophageal intraluminal lesion causing upper esophageal distension

Esophageal Distension

There are two main causes of diffuse esophageal distension:

- Esophageal motility disorders (achalasia, scleroderma, systemic lupus erythematosus, alcoholic neuropathy, anticholinergic drug use, esophagitis, etc.);
- Distal obstruction (benign or malignant stenosis, extrinsic mass-induced compression). A CT scan is useful to demonstrate a thickening of the wall secondary to tumor infiltration (pseudoachalasia) or extrinsic compression.

In esophageal motility disorders, the wall thickness should be normal; however, in certain cases there can be a symmetrical thickening at the gastroesophageal junction as a consequence of an inadequate distension, previous dilation procedures, myotomy, or esophagitis. This can make the differentiation from a tumor infiltration difficult.

Anterior Intestinal Cysts

Mediastinal cysts that originate from the anterior intestine constitute up to 10% of primary mediastinal masses. Mediastinal cysts are the consequence of embryologic aberrations and abnormal development of the primitive anterior intestine and of the primitive bronchial tree. The spectrum of bronchopulmonary malformations includes:

- Bronchogenic cysts: they are the most common intrathoracic cysts of the anterior intestine and are located, in order of frequency, in the carinal region, paratracheal region, esophageal wall, and retrocardiac region.
- Esophageal duplication cysts: they are usually located along the esophagus in the inferior portion of the posterior mediastinum.
- Neurenteric cysts: they communicate with the meninges and are associated to spine anomalies as butterfly vertebrae, hemivertebrae, and scoliosis.

Fatty Masses

Bochdalek Hernia

A Bochdalek hernia is a posterolateral diaphragmatic congenital defect that results in the persistence of the pleuroperitoneal canal. It is located on the left side in 90% of cases, due to the early closure of the right pleuroperitoneal canal and the relative protection provided by the liver. The organs involved in the herniation may be the stomach, the small or large intestine, the omentum or the kidney. On CT scans, a small Bochdalek hernia with fat content is observed in about 6% of patients.

Mediastinal Lipomatosis

Mediastinal lipomatosis is a deposition of adipose tissue in the mediastinum secondary to Cushing disease, high dose steroid therapy, or obesity. The infiltration may be located in the anterior mediastinum, close to the azygos vein and the aorta, but also in the paravertebral region and in the extrapleural space adjacent to the ribs.

Neurogenic Tumors

Neurogenic tumors usually present as masses in the posterior mediastinum, mainly in the paravertebral space along the intercostal and sympathetic nerves. They can be subdivided into three categories:

- Tumors from peripheral nerves (schwannomas 32% and neurofibromas 10%), more common among adults (Fig. 6.9)
- Tumors from sympathetic ganglia (ganglioneuromas 25%, ganglioneuroblastomas 14%, and neuroblastomas 15%), more common among pediatric patients
- Tumors from paraganglia (paragangliomas and chemodectomas 4%)

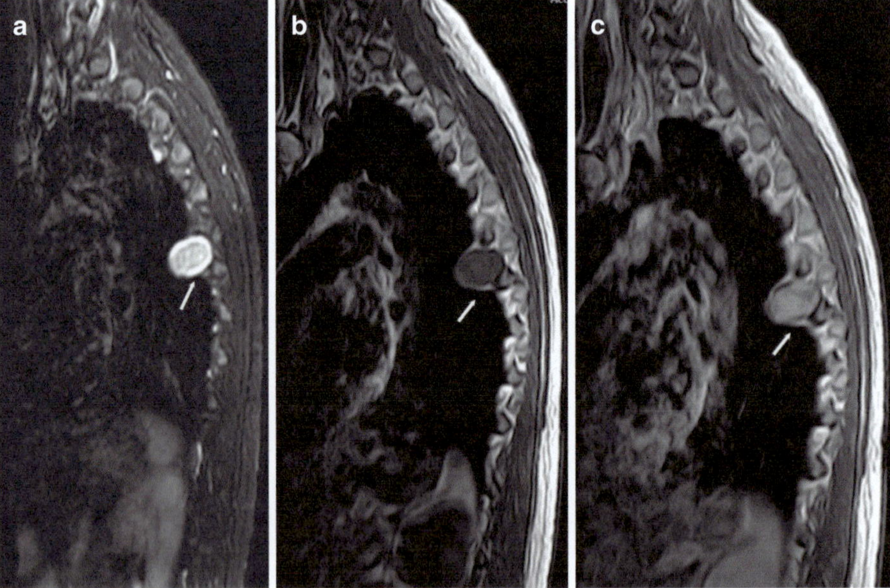

Fig. 6.9 Example of Schwannoma: the lesion is hyperintense in T2-weighted sequences (**a**, *arrow*) and enhances after contrast administration (**b** and **c**, *arrow*)

Neurogenic tumors may show an intraspinal extension, causing an enlargement of the neural foramen or the erosion of the adjacent rib. Calcifications might be present; if malignant, the tumor margins may often be poorly defined.

On CT scans, tumors from the peripheral nerves have lower attenuation than the muscles of the adjacent thoracic wall due to the high lipid content present in nervous tissue, interstitial fluid, and cystic degeneration. Enhancement after contrast administration does not allow to distinguish a benign from a malignant lesion.

A particular variant is plexiform neurofibromatosis that presents as an infiltrating mass involving the mediastinum along the distribution of the sympathetic chains, phrenic, recurrent laryngeal and vagus nerves.

Infectious Spondylitis

Staphylococcus aureus and other Gram-positive bacteria are the main pathogens responsible for infections of the axial skeleton. Tubercular spondylitis is probably the most common form of musculoskeletal tuberculosis. Fungal infections, such as coccidioidomycosis, can mimic tuberculosis both clinically and radiographically. A CT scan of infectious spondylitis shows a diffuse or focal involvement of the paravertebral soft tissues and an osteolytic vertebral destruction with or without marginal sclerosis. If the infection is caused by pyogenic bacteria, air bubbles can be observed within the bone or soft tissues.

Vertebral Column Tumors

Primary or metastatic tumors of the vertebral column usually arise in the vertebral body and can infiltrate the paravertebral space appearing as paravertebral masses. A CT scan shows the involvement of the posterior elements of the spine with the concomitant presence of osteoblastic or osteolytic bone lesions.

Spine Trauma

In case of trauma, CT plays an important role in evaluating the posterior mediastinal structures, paravertebral hematoma, and bone fragments in the spinal canal. Furthermore, it is a useful imaging modality for classifying the lesions and determining the site for surgical decompression.

Extramedullary Hematopoiesis

It occurs in some types of chronic hemolytic anemia (e.g., thalassemia, hereditary spherocytosis, homozygous sickle cell anemia) or in cases of massive bone marrow substitution by carcinomas or lymphomas. CT scans show unilateral or bilateral paravertebral masses that are often lobular, located along the lower thoracic spine, without erosion of the vertebral body. The presence of typical bone alterations can help in the diagnosis of thalassemia or sickle cell anemia.

Suggested Readings

Ackman JB. MR imaging of mediastinal masses. Magn Reson Imaging Clin N Am. 2015;23(2):141–64.

Jeung MY, et al. Imaging of cystic masses of the mediastinum. Radiographics. 2002;22:S79–93.

Thacker PG, et al. Imaging evaluation of mediastinal masses in children and adults: practical diagnostic approach based on a new classification system. J Thorac Imaging. 2015;30(4):247–67.

Whitten CR, et al. A diagnostic approach to mediastinal abnormalities. Radiographics. 2007;27(3):657–71.

Pulmonary Findings After Surgery, Radiotherapy, and Chemotherapy

7

Fabrizio Boni and Miriam Patella

In the diagnostic and therapeutic evaluation of patients who underwent lung surgery and/or radio-chemotherapy, imaging plays a key role in assessing the efficacy of therapy and identifying early or late complications. A CXR is mainly indicated for the early post-surgical evaluation to identify the presence of procedure-related pathological findings, such as pleural effusion, pneumothorax, or pneumonia; it also allows to evaluate the position of intrathoracic devices (drainages, vascular catheters, etc.). Instead, CT is preferred for the assessment of complex peri- and post-procedural complications and for the evaluation of the response to surgery or radio-chemotherapy. For a correct diagnosis, the radiologist has to have a vast technical knowledge of the surgical procedures, the mechanisms of action of the main chemotherapeutic drugs, and the modern applications of radiotherapy. Moreover, one has to be able to distinguish the "normal" radiological findings after these procedures from their complications.

Lung Surgery

Thoracic surgery includes a wide number of procedures, such as pneumonectomies (intrapleural, extrapleural, intrapericardial, and sleeve pneumonectomy), lobectomies, limited anatomical resections (sleeve lobectomy, segmentectomy), and non-anatomical resections (sleeve resection). Depending on the approach, these can be performed as open surgeries, requiring a sternotomy or a thoracotomy, or as minimally invasive interventions requiring thoracoscopy.

F. Boni (✉)
Department of Radiological, Oncological and Pathological Sciences, Sapienza University of Rome, Rome, Italy

M. Patella
Department of Thoracic Surgery, San Giovanni Hospital, EOC, Bellinzona, Switzerland
e-mail: miriam.patella@uniroma1.it

I. Carbone, M. Anzidei (eds.), *Thoracic Radiology*,
https://doi.org/10.1007/978-3-030-35765-8_7

Pneumonectomy

The intrapleural approach is the most commonly employed and consists in the resection of the lung and the visceral pleura. Extrapleural pneumonectomy includes the en bloc resection of the lung, parietal and mediastinal pleura, pericardium, and diaphragm. Intrapericardial pneumonectomy is the surgical removal of the lung with ligation of the intrapericardial portion of the pulmonary artery and/or vein. The infiltrated pericardium is also removed, and the resulting pericardial defect is closed with a synthetic mesh. This intrapericardial approach is indicated when the pathological tissue invades the hilum, and therefore a resection of the pericardium becomes necessary to remove all the tumor tissue and/or the region of pericardium involved. Sleeve pneumonectomy is an aggressive procedure that is indicated in case of bronchial tumors extending to the carina or to the distal portion of the trachea. After the resection, the anatomical continuity is restored by an end-to-end anastomosis that can be covered with protective flaps.

A patient's anatomy will be drastically changed by a pneumonectomy. Therefore, it is important to be familiar with the variations seen on imaging and their evolution in time to immediately recognize possible complications and to avoid the interpretation of normal findings as pathological. A CXR is a valid option for patient follow-up after pneumonectomy. In the first phases, typical findings are a **medially positioned trachea**, **mild contralateral hilar congestion**, and a **surgical cavity filled with fluids and air**. The amount of air that will accumulate is extremely variable; generally, during the first 4–5 days about half of the hemithorax will be filled, with a typical air-fluid level observable after a week. Then, a mediastinal ipsilateral shift to the operated side will occur due to the compensatory overexpansion of the contralateral lung and the gradual absorption of gases accumulated in the surgical cavity that will continue in the following weeks, with resulting progressive shift. The cavity will usually disappear over the next weeks or months, the heart rotates posteriorly, and the contralateral lung herniates across the midline and takes position anteriorly to the heart and the aorta. Therefore, a rapid mediastinal shift toward the remaining lung immediately after surgery is to be regarded as pathological and highly suggestive of atelectasis of the contralateral lung or a massive collection of gas and/or fluid within the cavity (due to a fistula, hemorrhage, or empyema). In later phases, a shift toward the residual parenchyma is suggestive of a late complication (Figs. 7.1 and 7.2).

Limited Anatomical Resections and Lobectomy

The primary aim of both limited resections and lobectomies is to preserve as much residual pulmonary function as possible while ensuring radical treatment. Limited anatomical resections (e.g., sleeve lobectomy, segmentectomy) and non-anatomical resections (e.g., sleeve resection) exist. The feasibility of the procedure and the choice of the appropriate intervention depend on the location and extent of the disease and on the clinical condition of the patient.

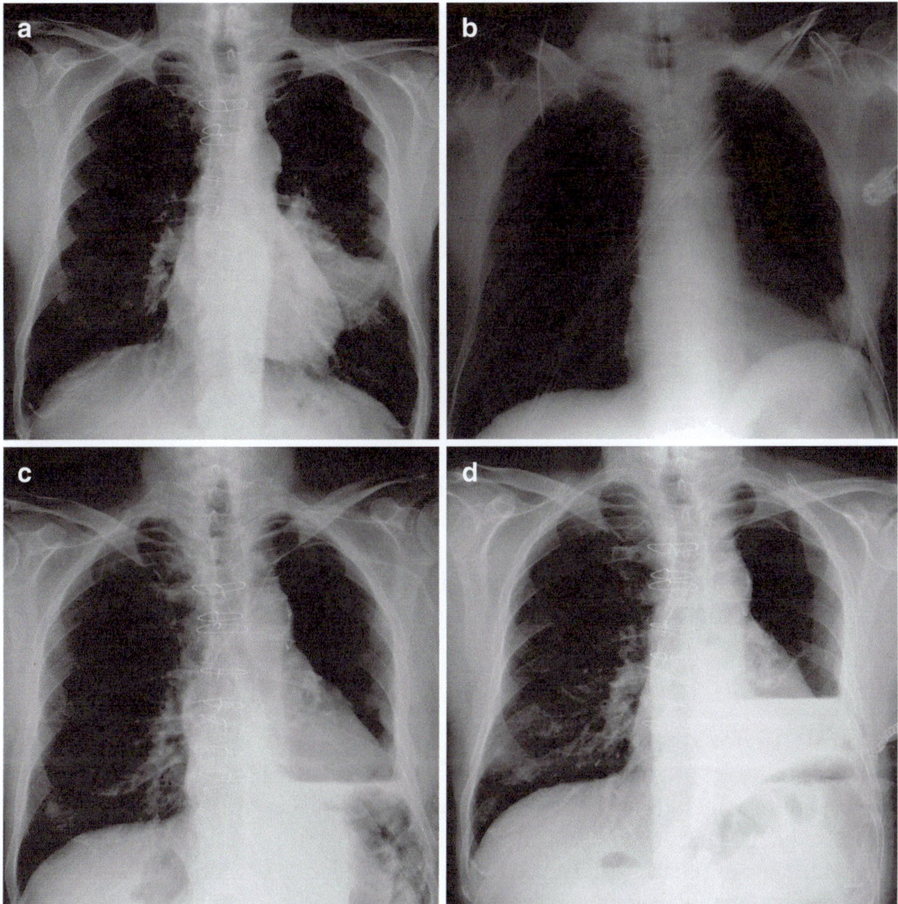

Fig. 7.1 (**a**) Chest X-ray before left pneumonectomy. (**b–d**) CXRs after the procedure. Immediate postoperative partial filling with fluid and air is observed on the treated hemithorax. Gradually, substitution of air with fluid and shift of the contralateral lung and mediastinum are observed in subsequent CXRs. A common early complication is hydropneumothorax with air-fluid level observed at the lower part of the left hemithorax (**c** and **d**)

A lobectomy consists in the resection of one lung lobe (or two lobes in case of bilobectomy), the afferent bronchovascular structures and the adjacent pleura. Mechanical staplers are used to avoid air leaks. Similarly, a segmentectomy involves the removal of the pulmonary segment affected and the affluent artery and bronchus. Apical, easier to access lung regions are more common to undergo segmentectomy.

Sleeve lobectomy provides an alternative to pneumonectomy in patients presenting with a bronchogenic carcinoma in a lobar orifice. En bloc resection of the lobe and a portion of the common airway is performed.

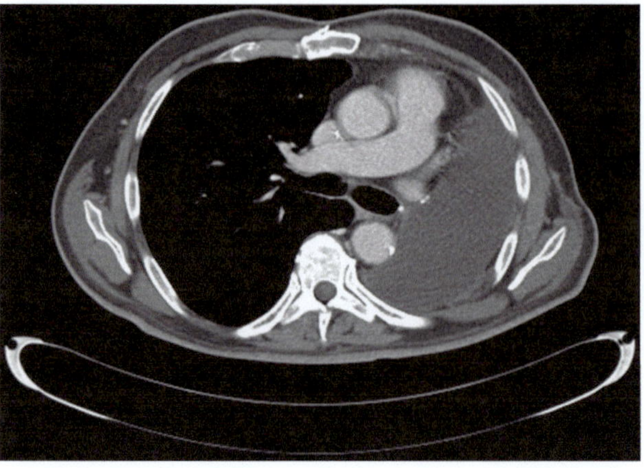

Fig. 7.2 Post left pneumonectomy CT scan with mediastinal shift and hyperinflation of the contralateral lung

Finally, a wedge resection is generally a V-shaped or U-shaped resection of a portion of the lung parenchyma that does not correspond to a lobar segment. The segmental bronchus and artery are typically preserved. Similarly to pneumonectomy, the normal anatomy is changed dramatically, though less evidently, by these approaches. A CXR remains a good instrument for the post-operatory assessment (Fig. 7.3).

Pleural Surgery

Pleural surgery includes a variety of interventions, among which pleurodesis is the most frequent. During this procedure, the pleural space is artificially obliterated after complete evacuation of the pleural fluid by induction of a sterile adhesive pleuritis. The indications for pleurodesis are recurrent pleural effusions, especially if neoplastic in origin, and recurrent pneumothorax. Based on the substance introduced between the visceral and parietal pleura, three different types of pleurodesis are recognized:

- Sclerosing: talc powder, bleomycin, doxycycline
- Cytostatic: cisplatin
- Mechanical: abrasion with Bovie scratch pads, used in young patients with benign disease.

Postoperative Complications

Knowing the normal postoperative course and its variations permits an easy recognition of possible complications. These, by definition, are divided into early and late.

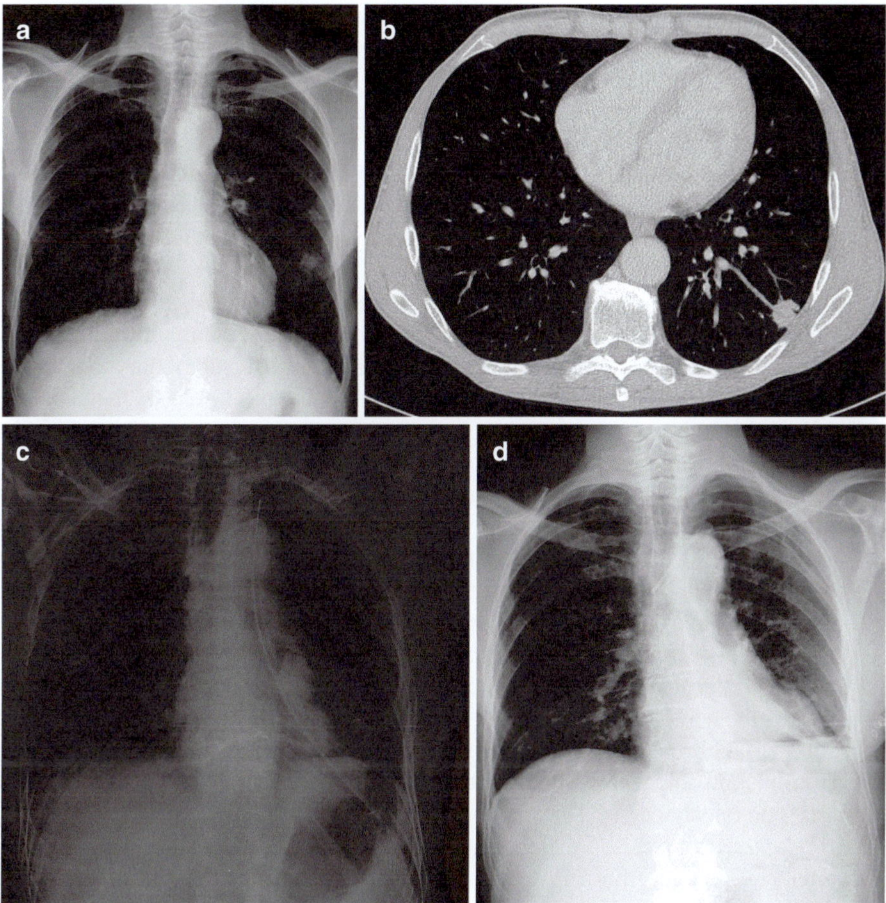

Fig. 7.3 CXR (**a**) and CT scan (**b**) before left inferior lobectomy, with the tumor adjacent to the pleura. (**c**) On postprocedural CXR, there is a drainage placed on the left; surgical clips and subcutaneous emphysema are also evident on the treated side. (**d**) Hydropneumothorax on the left lung is evident, with air-fluid level and obliteration of the costodiaphragmatic recess

Early Complications

1. *Pulmonary edema*: a potentially lethal condition that can occur after pneumonectomy, with a prevalence of 2.5–5% (less frequently after bilobectomy, <1% after lobectomy) and an 80–100% mortality rate. The pathogenesis is not completely clear though it is known that an increase of the hydrostatic pressure and an altered capillary permeability play a predominant role. Among the contributing causes are over-hydration during the procedure, left ventricular failure, hypoproteinemia, leakage syndrome, and prolonged exposure to high oxygen concentrations. Patients undergoing a right pneumonectomy have a higher probability to develop pulmonary edema. This is probably due to the

accumulation of fluid in the surgical cavity causing an increase in blood flow in the left lung, which normally receives only 45% of the cardiac output and contains about 45% of the pulmonary lymphatic system.

When a patient rapidly develops dyspnea and hypoxia, postpneumonectomy pulmonary edema is a clinical and radiological diagnosis of exclusion after ruling out other infectious causes (including aspiration pneumonia), thromboembolism, bronchopleural fistula, and other causes of ARDS. In the most severe cases, serial CXRs will show typical parenchymal opacities that are identical to those observed in other forms of ARDS. In less severe cases, the typical CXR findings of pulmonary edema with Kerley lines, peribronchial cuffing, and perihilar haze are present. If a CT scan becomes necessary, the main findings will be interlobular septal thickening, cuffing, and diffuse pulmonary opacities. Pleural effusion will present only if the accumulated fluid exceeds the capacity of lymphatic drainage.

2. *Hemothorax*: in the immediate postoperative period, small amounts of blood can normally be present secondary to the lesion of small vessels during the procedure. Instead, more voluminous bleedings represent a feared complication and are due to insufficient hemostasis of a bronchial artery or of the thoracic wall or, in much rarer cases, due to bleeding from a ligated pulmonary artery. Even in cases of uncontrolled bleeding the mortality is low (<0.1%). A hemothorax typically presents as a rapidly evolving pleural effusion. On CT, the increased density of the effusion can be appreciated both in quality and quantity. As the hemothorax has the tendency to coagulate, pseudomasses formed by subpleural fibrin deposits can occur. Nevertheless, these are easily distinguished from pleural thickenings due to other causes by their higher Hounsfield Units (HU) on unenhanced CT scans.
3. *Chylothorax*: it refers to the accumulation of lymphatic fluid in the pleural space after a lesion to the thoracic duct or one of its main branches. A typical radiological finding is the rapid filling of the pleural space after pneumonectomy though it does not allow to differentiate chylothorax from other causes of effusions. The CT scan does not allow a definitive diagnosis of the nature of the effusion as chylothorax can present with different densities. The presence of multiloculated effusions can be an important suggestive finding. The gold-standard diagnostic test is lymphangiography, even if a certain diagnosis is also possible when considering the laboratory tests (triglycerides level >110 mg/dL).
4. *Bronchopleural fistula (BPF)*: a potentially lethal complication, with a prevalence of 2–13% and a mortality rate of 16–23%. The main cause of death in these patients is generally the occurrence of aspiration pneumonia with consequent ARDS. It is more common after a right rather than a left pneumonectomy due to the different anatomical characteristics of the right bronchus, mainly the different caliber. It can occur as an early complication in case of suture dehiscence, or as a late complication when consequent to a recurrence or a perianastomotic infection. The radiological signs of a BPF can be: steady increase in intrapleural air space, air-fluid level formation or changes in a pre-existing air-fluid level, development of tension pneumothorax, drop in the air-fluid level of

more than 1.5–2 cm within the surgical cavity. Therefore, it is of critical importance to monitor the changes in the air-fluid levels after a pneumonectomy, as the increase of air and a decrease of the fluid are important signs of a BPF. HRCT is fundamental in these patients both for diagnosis and for treatment planning: multiplanar reconstructions often allow direct visualization of the fistulous tract between the bronchial lumen and the surgical cavity.

5. *Empyema*: a serious but infrequent complication, with an incidence of 2–16% and a mortality of 16–71%. It is more frequent when a pneumonectomy is performed after a previous lobectomy. Mortality is increased when it is associated to a BPF. Though it tends to be an early complication, it can occur even months or years after the intervention. On CXR, empyema presents with multiple air-fluid levels within the cavity; these findings may be absent initially, making the CXR inconclusive. CT is a more sensitive test for patients with suspected empyema, showing an enlargement of the surgical cavity (behavior similar to an expansive process). Other signs are:
   (a) complicated effusion
   (b) irregular thickening of the residual parietal pleura and enhancement of the wall after intravenous contrast administration
   (c) convexity or partial loss of the normal concavity of the mediastinal contour of the cavity, evidence of a BPF (eventually associated)
6. *Persistent air leak*: after a lobectomy or a segmentectomy, virtually all patients will have a mild postoperative air leak (especially when there are incomplete or absent fissures) that tends to resolve spontaneously. With more significant air leaks, the CXR and CT will show persistent pneumothorax with or without a pneumomediastinum or subcutaneous emphysema. Almost all the leaks that originate in the peripheral regions of the lung are self-limited within 24–48 h, when the residual parenchyma completely fills the pleural cavity. A leak is defined as persistent when still present on the seventh postoperative day. Nevertheless, this condition has not a significant impact on the postoperative mortality.
7. *ARDS*: a lethal complication with a prevalence of about 5% (after pneumonectomies) and a mortality rate of 80% (compared to 65% in ARDS in non-operated patients). When the clinical presentation is suggestive, ARDS is diagnosed by serial CXRs that show the rapid appearance of diffuse opacities in the residual parenchyma. On CT, there will be ground-glass opacifications and interlobular septal thickening with the development of the lesions following an anteroposterior gradient. ARDS can develop alone or in combination with other complications like pneumonia or BPF with or without empyema.
8. *Pneumonia*: has a prevalence between 2 and 22% after thoracotomy and a mortality rate of up to 25%. Aspiration of gastric secretions and bacterial colonization of the atelectatic pulmonary parenchyma are the most common etiologies. Predisposing factors (especially for aspiration pneumonia) are intubation and invasive ventilation. In surgical patients, the signs, symptoms and radiological presentation may sometimes lead to an over-diagnosis of postoperative pneumonia. On the other hand, the opposite error (unrecognized pneumonia) may be

fatal. Additional difficulties result from the consideration that, on some occasions, a negative CXR cannot rule out pneumonia with certainty as this may become radiologically visible only later, after the first symptoms appear. The general radiological presentation can vary from foci of increased opacity, to bronchopneumonia, to lobar pneumonia (less common). Aspiration pneumonia can evolve into necrotizing forms with formation of abscesses.

9. *Gossypiboma*: this term is used to describe the formation of granulation tissue around a foreign body such as a retained surgical gauze. Most commonly, it occurs in the pleural space, but sometimes the mass can invaginate within the pulmonary parenchyma, simulating a parenchymal lesion. CT will show a mass frequently with capsular enhancement and a central hyperdensity. Often, air can be present at the center of the lesion. During the early postoperative course, the mass can be radiologically confused with an abscess, a loculated empyema, a complicated hematoma or a seroma. In later stages, the differential diagnoses include chronic infections, granulomatous processes, neoformations.
10. *Atelectasis*: can result from an incomplete ventilation of the residual parenchyma after partial lung resections. It occurs in about 5–10% of sleeve resections as a consequence of the formation of edema at the anastomotic site, the interruption of the ciliated epithelium and lymphatic vessels or a partial denervation of the lobe. On CT, there will be ground-glass opacifications or consolidations in the atelectatic region.
11. *Others*: less frequent early complications worth of mention are lung torsion, cardiac herniation, and anastomotic dehiscence (Figs. 7.4, 7.5, 7.6, and 7.7).

Late Complications

1. *Postpneumonectomy syndrome*: is a late complication caused by an excessive compensatory response after a lung resection with a consequent compression of the main intrathoracic airways. Young and more responsive patients will be affected more often. The bronchial stenosis causes stridor that can be assessed on the physical examination and can predispose to the development of infections. The CXR can show a shift of the trachea, mediastinum, and heart toward the surgical cavity. CT and bronchoscopy can provide an optimal visualization of the airway compression. The former also adds precise information about the site of bronchial obstruction.
2. *Esophageal-pleural fistula*: is a devastating complication occurring in about 0.2–1% of the patients after pneumonectomy. It can occur as an early complication (secondary to an iatrogenic damage or the compression of the arterial supply), but more commonly is a late complication due to chronic inflammation at the level of the esophagus or of the perianastomotic region or due to disease recurrence. CXR is often not sufficient for a diagnosis; the esophagography can visualize the fistula. CT is the gold-standard as it visualizes the fistula, the underlying cause, and any associated empyema.
3. *Bronchial anastomotic stenosis*: is the most common complication after sleeve resection (more than 18% of patients) and can be potentially very serious. It is due to the interruption of the vascular supply to the distal bronchial segment that

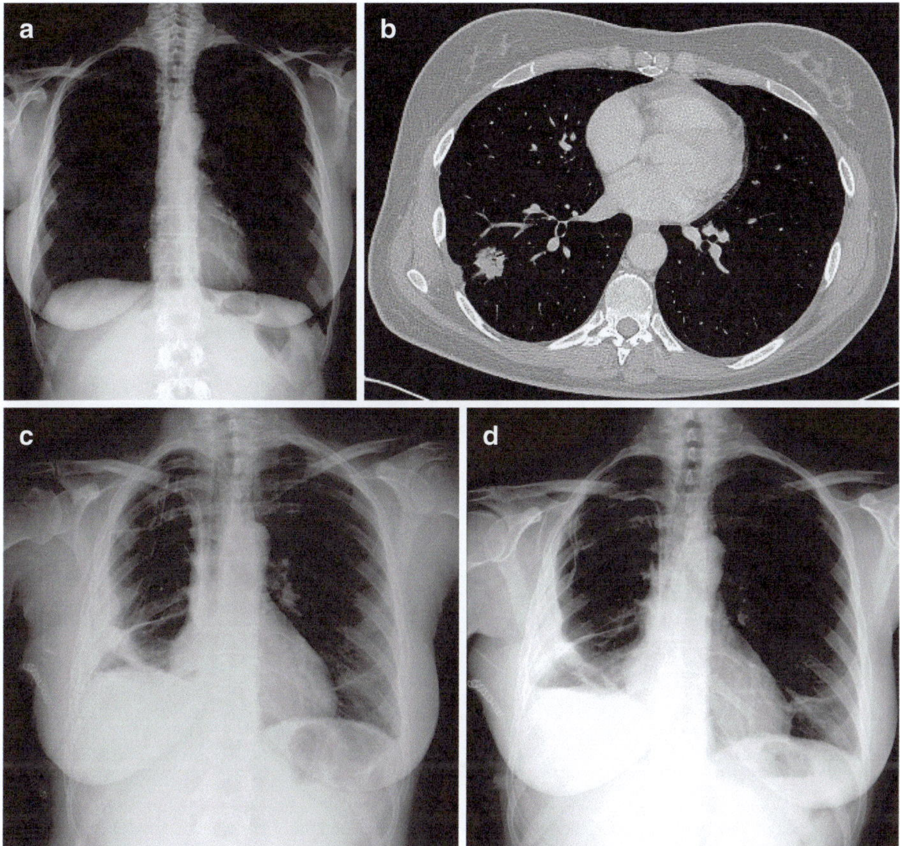

Fig. 7.4 (**a**, **b**) The lesion on the lateral basal segment of the right inferior lobe was treated with a right inferior lobectomy. (**c**) On postoperative CXR, the surgical clips, the drainage, and the central venous catheter are present in the right hemithorax. On the right inferior lung field, an intrascissural fibrotic process is visible with an air-fluid level immediately below: this is an example of hemopneumothorax (**c**, **d**)

results into a partial anastomotic dehiscence with formation of granulation tissue. The CT is more precise than CXR in identifying the anastomotic stenosis.

4. *Infections*: can present as BPF or pleural empyema but are generally much less common than early infections.
5. *Recurrence*: may result from an incomplete resection of the pathology, ipsilateral mediastinal lymphadenopathies, recurrences in the thoracic wall or parietal pleura, positive surgical margins (that are possible even with adequate margins, negative at the histological exam). The CT is the standard of care to evaluate recurrences. Nevertheless, it may be difficult to distinguish not well-defined small recurrences without the shift of surrounding structures from postoperative fibrosis. In these cases, a bronchoscopy and a PET-CT may be helpful, as well as serial monitoring during follow-up.

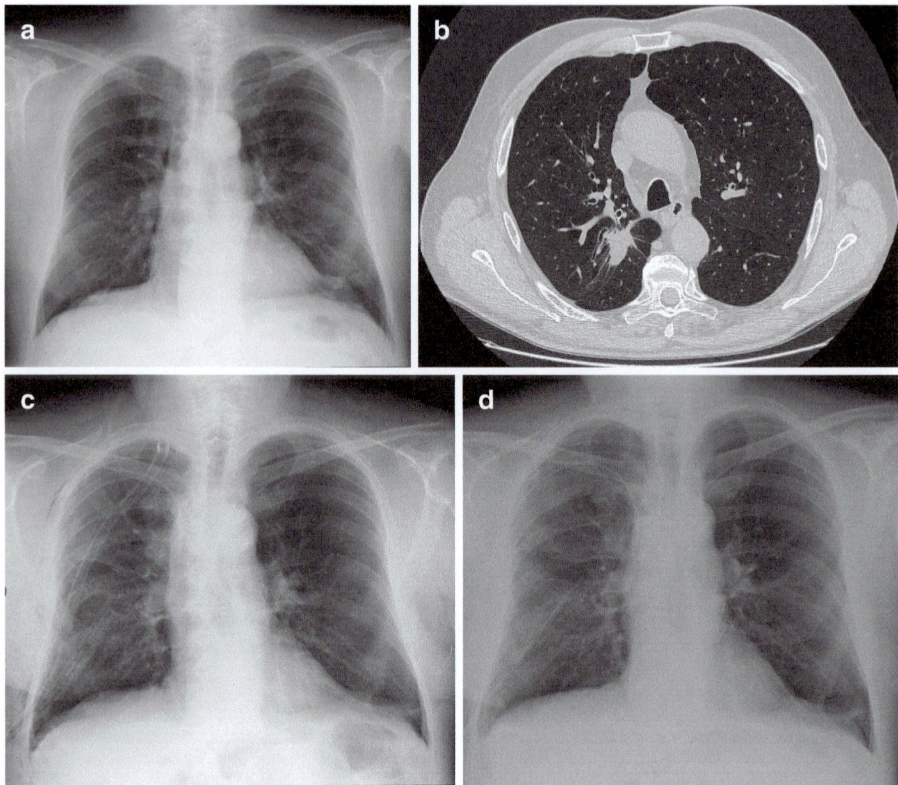

Fig. 7.5 Chest X-ray (**a**) and CT scan (**b**) acquired before atypical right superior lobe resection. (**c**) On postprocedural CXR, a drainage and subcutaneous emphysema is present. (**d**) The second postoperative day, this patient developed a chylothorax with increased opacity of the right hemithorax

Fig. 7.6 (**a**, **b**) Pre-right lobectomy CT scan and CXR with a lesion evident in the superior segment of the right lower lobe. (**c**) CXR immediately after the procedure with a drainage and a central venous catheter visible on the right. The inferior right lobe removed is replaced with fluid and air. Subcutaneous emphysema is visible immediately after the surgical clips on the right. (**d**, **e**) The subcutaneous emphysema worsened, expanding upward and to the other side; therefore, a drainage was placed under fluoroscopic guidance. (**f**, **g**) Subsequent CXRs demonstrate improvement and resolution of this complication. Upward shift of the diaphragm on the right side is appreciated (**g**)

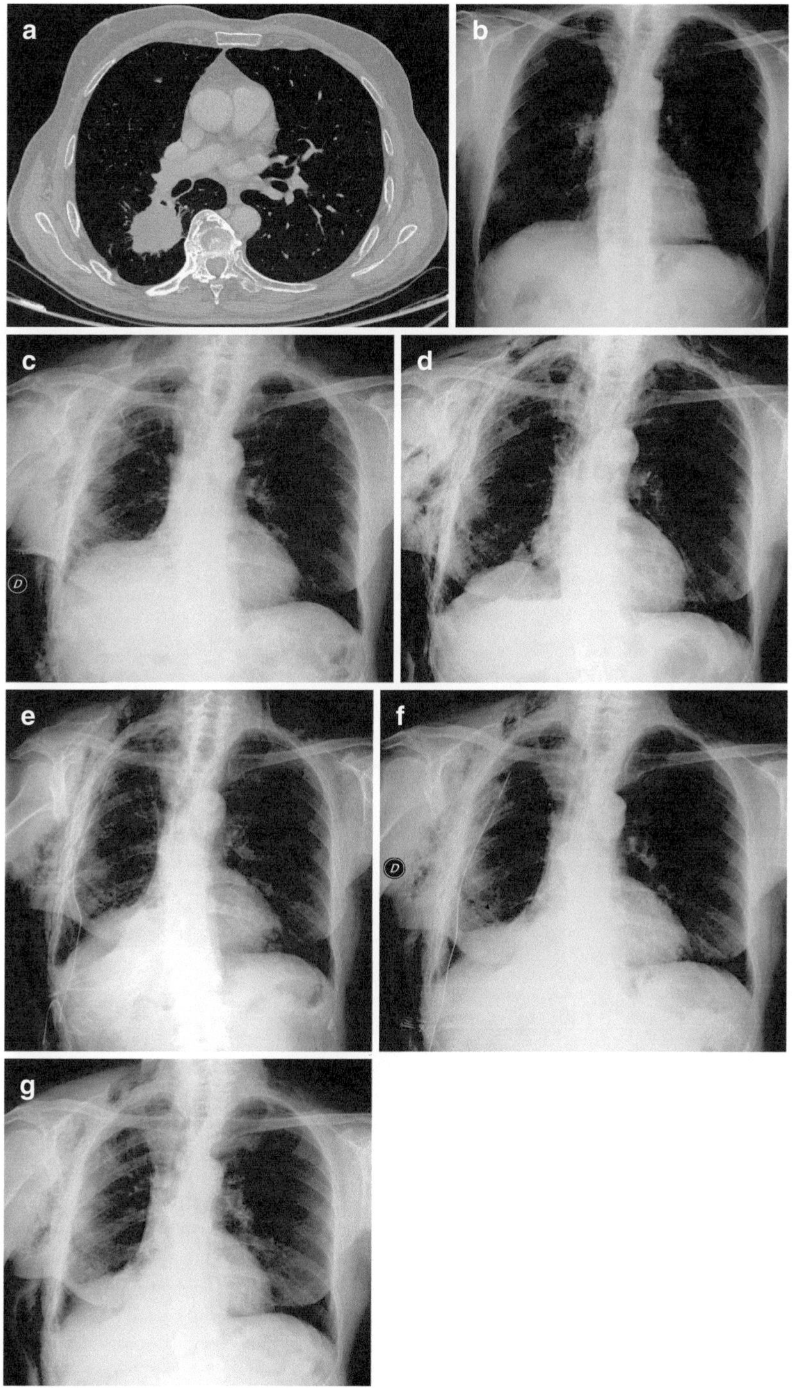
a
b
c
d
e
f
g

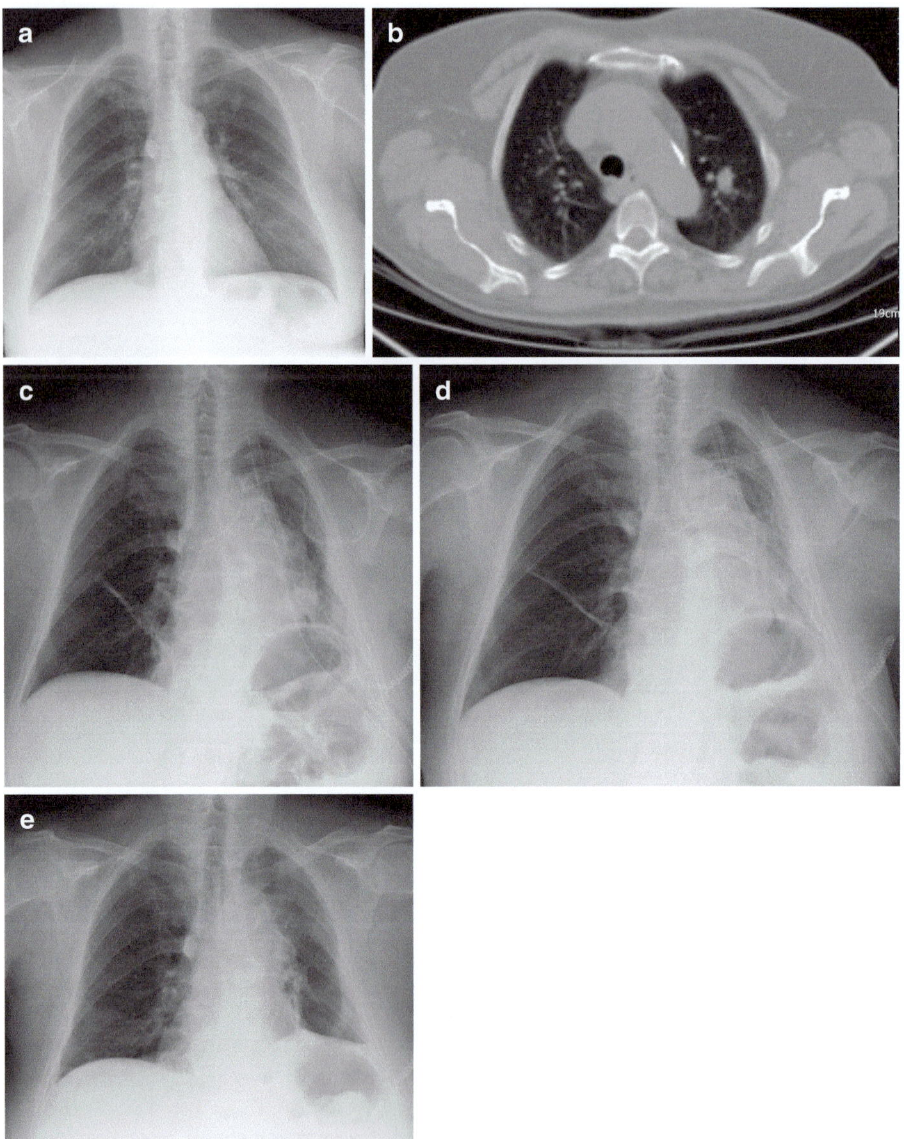

Fig. 7.7 (**a**, **b**) Pre-operative CXR and CT scan showing a superior left lung lesion. (**c**) Immediately post-procedure, the surgical clips, a drainage, and a central venous catheter are observed on the left side. The elevation of the left hemidiaphragm is accompanied by the mediastinal shift towards the treated side. An apical pneumothorax is visible. (**d**) After 5 days from surgery, atelectasis of the left inferior lobe developed and can be appreciated as a region of increased opacity. (**f**) A fibrotic process developed on the treated side, at the inferior lung field. The left costophrenic angle is obliterated

Radiotherapy on the Lung

Radiotherapy (RT) is a possible treatment for lung cancer with curative (stage I-II, inoperable for other reasons), adjuvant or neoadjuvant (stage IIIa), or palliative intent. The historical radiotherapy regimens used to deliver significant radiations to regions of the lung beyond the margins of the pathology. This entailed a high risk of radiation-induced damage of the surrounding healthy pulmonary parenchyma (Radiation-Induced Lung Disease, RILD). Nowadays, new techniques have been developed to reduce the toxic effects of delivered radiations. 3D-Conformal Radiation Therapy (CRT) and Stereotactic Body Radiotherapy (SBRT) use multiple radiation beams that distribute the dose strictly within the target. Despite the improvements with these techniques, the possibility of a radiation-induced parenchymal damage is still a real risk in patients undergoing radiotherapy for neoplasia in any part of the thoracic district. The risk is strictly correlated to the radiation dose, the tumor site, and patient-specific factors (e.g., concurrent chemotherapy treatment: drugs like actinomycin D, busulfan, or bleomycin can worsen the radiation-induced damage). There is no linear correlation between the radiation dose and the damage, but generally there is a cut-off above which the prevalence is increased. It is uncommon to have any parenchymal damage with a total radiation dose inferior to 20 Gy (sub-lethal dose) while it is common with 30–40 Gy and is basically always present with a dose superior to 40 Gy.

The toxic effects of radiotherapy are summarized in Table 7.1.

Table 7.1 Possible presentations of radiotherapy-induced damage

	Timing	Clinical presentation	Pattern	HRCT findings
Very early effects	Hours/days after radiotherapy (immediate)	Asymptomatic	Pulmonary edema Exudative alveolitis Hypersecretion	None
Radiation pneumonitis	3–6 months after radiotherapy (acute)	Moderate/severe dyspnea Non-productive cough (60%) Low-grade fever (10%)	Respiratory failure Pulmonary hypertension	Lesions confined to the treated area: – Ground glass – Parenchymal consolidations
Radiation-induced fibrosis	6 months/years after radiotherapy (chronic)	Asymptomatic or dyspnea of variable severity	Chronic respiratory failure	– Parenchymal consolidation with air bronchogram, loss of volume, and atelectasis – Pseudomass: loss of volume and consolidation – Linear pseudo-scarring fibrosis

Radiation-induced toxicity can cause lung damage very early; in addition, we can recognize two more distinct clinical, pathological, and radiological presentations based on the time of onset. Early radiation pneumonia usually occurs within 1–6 months after ending the treatment. Chronic radiation fibrosis is a chronic phase occurring 6 and 12 months after ending therapy.

Acute Pulmonary Damage

Radiological findings of acute pulmonary damage after a standard radiotherapy regimen are ground-glass opacifications, parenchymal consolidation, or both (usually in the lung that has been irradiated). Occasionally, ipsilateral pleural effusion and atelectasis can occur during radiation pneumonitis. With the introduction of new techniques such as CRT and SBRT, the presentation of radiation-induced pulmonary damage has changed and knowing the kind of treatment the patient underwent is of fundamental importance when interpreting the radiological images. Since these techniques deliver the radiation dose to the tumor through multiple radiation beams, any radiation-induced damage will be different in morphology, characteristics, localization, extension, and distribution compared to classical radiotherapy.

CRT- or SBRT-induced damages are described as unusual or atypical. After CRT, radiation pneumonitis can present as focal or nodular ground-glass opacifications, parenchymal consolidation, or both. The findings are limited to the treated tumor and to the immediately adjacent healthy parenchyma; nevertheless, damage distant from the lesion and/or in the contralateral lung has also been reported in the literature. Usually, after SBRT no damage occurs distantly from the treated site. Thanks to the sharp dose gradient between the boundaries of the target area (high-dose area) and the surrounding healthy tissues (low-dose area), the post-SBRT damages are usually confined to the treated region and trace the shape of the lesion. This type of radiation-induced damage has been classified by Ikezoe into four patterns:

- diffuse consolidation
- diffuse ground-glass opacities
- patchy consolidation and ground-glass opacities
- patchy ground-glass opacities

Chronic Pulmonary Fibrosis

Usually, the typical findings of radiation pneumonitis after conventional RT treatment gradually resolve within the next 6 months. When the damage is limited, there are no radiological sequelae, but with more extended damages a progression to fibrosis is common. The radiological presentation of chronic pulmonary fibrosis is a well-delimited area of volume loss with a linear scar or a parenchymal consolidation. Parenchymal distortion and traction bronchiectasis can also be observed. In time, the fibrosis can either stabilize or progress for more than 24 months.

Progression of damage can also appear as a reduction in size of the fibrotic parenchymal consolidation or the appearance of a sharp demarcation from the normal parenchyma. Occasionally, an ipsilateral mediastinal shift and an adjacent pleural thickening/effusion can also be present.

Chronic pulmonary fibrosis after CRT and SBRT can present with one of three different patterns:

- The **conventional modified pattern** consists in a well-demarcated parenchymal consolidation area with volume loss and traction bronchiectasis. Its name is derived from its similarity with the pattern observed after conventional radiotherapy, from which it differs mainly for the smaller extension.
- The **mass-like pattern** is derived from the previous one. The pattern is defined mass-like when the alterations described above are focal and confined to a 2 cm margin around the treated lesion. Usually, the mass-like alteration appears bigger in size than the original treated lesion.
- The **scar-like pattern** consists in a linear opacity, <1 cm wide, associated with moderate/severe volume loss. This finding persists in the treated tumor site even when the lesion is completely (or almost completely) resolved. This is the pattern that differs the most from the typical presentation after conventional RT.

Differential Diagnosis

A definitive diagnosis of radiation-induced pneumonitis is difficult to make as its presentation may be clinically and radiologically equal to an infection or a disease recurrence. To improve the diagnostic accuracy, it is of fundamental importance to know the timing, type, and dose of radiotherapy.

- **Pneumonia**: the possibility of an infection should be considered when a CT scan shows pulmonary opacities before the end of radiotherapy or diffuse or bilateral parenchymal anomalies. The presence of centrilobular nodules is another suggestive sign of infection, indicating bronchiolar processes (tree-in-bud), and is sometimes associated to consolidations or cavitations (common in case of tuberculosis). Occasionally, a superinfection can complicate the radiation-induced toxicity and in these cases cavitations are common. Keep in mind that the course of radiation-induced pneumonitis is more indolent than infectious pneumonia. Therefore, a sudden onset of symptoms and a sudden appearance of radiological findings is more suggestive of an infectious etiology.
- **Carcinomatous lymphangitis**: causes dyspnea, mimicking the clinical presentation of radiotherapy-induced damage. However, a higher severity and more rapid progression of symptoms are suggestive of lymphangitis; it is also associated to irregular thickening of the interlobular septa, peribronchial cuffing, pleural effusion, and mediastinal lymphadenopathies.
- **Recurrence**: usually occurs within 2 years after therapy and depends on the size of the treated lesion, its stage, its histotype, and the type of previous treatment. A

Table 7.2 Possible effects of radiation-induced extrapulmonary toxicity

Site	Alteration
Thymus	Thymic cysts
Lymph nodes	Diffuse calcifications (indicative of treatment response)
Heart	Pericardial effusion Chronic pericarditis Valvular heart disease
Esophagus	Motility disorders Strictures
Bones	Rib fractures Osteitis
Muscles	Myositis

diagnosis of recurrence is often very difficult to make on CT scans of patients who developed radiation fibrosis, especially if occurring in a mass-like pattern.

– A typical CT sign of stable radiation fibrosis is lung consolidation with regular margins and air bronchograms. Locoregional recurrences tend to cause an alteration of the contours and/or the dimensions of the fibrotic area, forming a homogeneous opacity without air bronchograms and with convex margins. The diagnosis is easier when other signs of disease recurrence are present, such as nodules in other sites of the ipsilateral or contralateral parenchyma, pleural effusion, mediastinal lymphadenopathies, etc. Sometimes, neither CXRs nor the CT or MRI allow a certain diagnosis between residual/recurrent disease and radiation-induced damage. In these cases, a 18-FDG PET scan is a valid option to distinguish the tumor tissue (metabolically active) from radiation fibrosis (metabolically inactive). Nevertheless, as the radiation-induced pneumonitis can lead to an increased FDG uptake that may be misinterpreted as a residual/recurrent disease, PET should be performed at least 3 months after the end of radiotherapy to reduce the risk of false positives to a minimum. Finally, it should be noted that in rare cases there may be an increased FDG uptake for up to 15 months after the end of radiotherapy even in the absence of tumor recurrence. In these cases, a biopsy becomes necessary.

Radiation Toxicity in Other Sites

Other alterations can occur in the thoracic structures of patients who underwent radiotherapy (lung or other sites, as mediastinum or breast). The main manifestations are summarized in Table 7.2.

Chemotherapy for the Lung

Chemotherapy has a key role in the management of patients with lung cancer, having an indication in all classes of patients as a neoadjuvant (stage IIIa and IIIb) or adjuvant (stage I, II, III) therapy. The traditional drugs are inhibitors of cell division and therefore target rapidly proliferating cells. New classes of drugs (target therapy) are directed toward specific molecules on the membrane or within the cell responsible for cellular activity. Cytotoxic chemotherapeutic drugs interfere with DNA and RNA synthesis or with cell division, altering cell growth through multiple mechanisms. The most common traditional drugs are: cyclophosphamide (alkylating agent), cisplatin (DNA-intercalating agent), fluorouracil (antimetabolite), doxorubicin (anthracycline), and bleomycin. Some more recent agents are worth of note: gemcitabine (antimetabolite), oxaliplatin (platinum analog), paclitaxel and docetaxel (taxanes, antifungal agents), and irinotecan (topoisomerase inhibitor). If the damage induced by the drug overcomes the repair capacity of the cell, necrosis, or apoptosis occur. The aim is to have a bigger effect on tumor tissue than on healthy tissue. With the increasing knowledge on the biology of tumors, molecular therapies have been developed: targets can be antigens (in case of monoclonal antibodies) or signaling molecules (in case of kinase inhibitors). In these groups, we find EGFR (a growth factor involved in the tumor proliferation) inhibitors, ALK (a membrane receptor that transmits growth signals to the cell) inhibitors and angiogenesis inhibitors (targeting VEGF). Finally, Nivolumab (an immunodrug) is the first and only PD-1 immune checkpoint inhibitor, currently used for squamous-cell non-small cell lung cancer as a second-line treatment. Tables 7.3 and 7.4 summarize the main classes of chemotherapeutic agents used for the treatment of lung cancer and their possible toxic effects on the lung parenchyma.

Knowing the main mechanisms of action of these drugs is important for two main reasons. First, it raises the accuracy in the evaluation of the response (or lack of response) to therapy. For example, it is important to know that when a patient is treated with an immunodrug, an increased dimension of the lesion at the first, early, follow-up may be an indication of a possible response to therapy (intratumoral immune response). Secondly, it allows prompt diagnosis (or at least a suspicion) of

Table 7.3 Main classes of chemotherapeutic agents used for lung cancer

Class	Agents
Platinum analogs	Cisplatin, carboplatin
Antimetabolites	Gemcitabine, pemetrexed
Vinca alkaloids	Vinorelbine
Taxanes	Docetaxel, paclitaxel
Topoisomerase inhibitors	Etoposide, topotecan
Tyrosine kinase inhibitors	Gefitinib, erlotinib, afatinib, crizotinib
PD-1 inhibitor	Nivolumab

Table 7.4 Possible presentations of toxic effects of chemotherapeutic drugs

Presentation	Drug
Pulmonary infiltrates	Bleomycin, methotrexate, gemcitabine, paclitaxel, oxaliplatin, everolimus/temsirolimus, gefitinib, erlotinib, rituximab
Pulmonary edema	All-trans retinoic acids, gemcitabine, interleukin 2, interferon
Pulmonary hemorrhage	Bevacizumab
Pericardial effusion	All-trans retinoic acids, imatinib

eventual adverse events. Indeed, if the toxic effects of the traditional drugs are somewhat expected, the toxic effects of the target therapies are less predictable.

Pulmonary Toxicity

When a patient is being treated with chemotherapy for lung cancer, pulmonary parenchymal alterations can occur because of toxic effects of the drug, infections, or underlying pathology. Among drug-induced alterations, different patterns can be recognized:

- *Pulmonary infiltrates*: can occur as early alterations, with parenchymal infiltrates, pulmonary edema and hypersensitivity reactions or pleural effusion, or as late alterations (2 months or more after therapy), with infiltrates and fibrosis. The toxicity of some old-generation drugs can be dose-dependent (cumulative dose with bleomycin and carmustine). On CT scan, we can differentiate four types of drug-induced pulmonary infiltrates:

  nonspecific areas of ground-glass opacities
  multiple parenchymal consolidations
  sparse ground-glass opacities with interlobular septal thickening
  diffuse bilateral ground-glass opacities, or parenchymal consolidations with traction bronchiectasis

  The most common pattern is the nonspecific areas of ground-glass opacities; the one associated to the highest mortality is the bilateral diffuse ground-glass opacities, indicative of diffuse alveolar damage.
- *Pulmonary hemorrhage*: is a potentially fatal complication described in patients with non-small cell lung cancer in therapy with bevacizumab (up to 5% incidence). The mechanism through which this drug causes the hemorrhage is not completely known, but some studies have identified as possible pre-treatment risk factors the presence of necrosis and/or intralesional cavitations. Moreover, this complication seems to be more common in squamous cells carcinoma, which therefore is an exclusion criterion for this treatment.
- *Capillary leak syndrome*: is caused by a sudden hyperpermeability with plasma extravasation from the intravascular to the extravascular space and is characterized by generalized edema, hypotension, dehydration, and hypoproteinemia. The radiological pattern is due to the increased vascular permeability that leads to fluid and proteins extravasation from the capillaries, basically presenting as an interstitial edema characterized by multiple and confluent ground-glass opacities. It frequently evolves into ARDS and noncardiogenic pulmonary edema. It is important to differentiate this complication from other forms of pulmonary toxicity because treatment of capillary leak syndrome requires the use of diuretics (in addition to the discontinuation of the drug and cortisone). Gemcitabine is the chemotherapeutic agent most commonly involved.

Suggested Readings

Chae EJ, et al. Radiographic and CT findings of thoracic complications after pneumonectomy. Radiographics. 2006;26:1449–67.

Diederich S, et al. Chest CT for suspected pulmonary complications of oncologic therapies: how I review and report. Cancer Imaging. 2016;16(1):7.

Kim EA, et al. Radiographic and CT findings in complications following pulmonary resection. Radiographics. 2002;22:67–86.

Larici AR, et al. Lung abnormalities at multimodality imaging after radiation therapy for non–small cell lung cancer. Radiographics. 2011;31:771–89.

Pneumonia and Bronchiolitis

8

Alessandro Maria Ferrazza and Paolo Baldassarri

Infections of the lower respiratory tract can remain localized to the airways (resulting in tracheitis, bronchitis, and bronchiolitis) or can reach the lung parenchyma (resulting in pneumonia). Even though a CXR is generally sufficient to establish the diagnosis of a pneumonic process, an HRCT becomes necessary in many cases, particularly if atypical processes or bronchiolar involvement occur.

Pneumonia

Pulmonary infections can be differentiated based on the location and pattern of the parenchymal involvement (Table 8.1).

When a CT scan is performed, it is possible to identify specific signs that help diagnose the etiology of the inflammatory process. The following radiological phenotypes are described:

- *Bacteria: Gram-positive cocci*
  - *Streptococcus pneumoniae*: the most common pathogen, responsible for about 40% of cases. It usually causes a typical lobar pneumonia but can present as bronchopneumonia in a minority of cases. Complications such as cavitation, gangrene, or pneumatoceles occur very rarely. Observed only in about 10% of cases, pleural effusion is infrequent as well.
  - *Staphylococcus aureus*: although responsible for only 3% of community-acquired pneumonias (CAPs), it is a frequent etiologic agent in hospital-acquired pneumonias (HAPs). The most common presentation is a segmental bronchopneumonia. The consolidations can be patchy or homogeneous when multiple foci coalesce. Atelectasis occurs frequently due to the involvement of

A. M. Ferrazza (✉) · P. Baldassarri
Department of Radiological, Oncological and Pathological Sciences, Sapienza University of Rome, Rome, Italy

I. Carbone, M. Anzidei (eds.), *Thoracic Radiology*,
https://doi.org/10.1007/978-3-030-35765-8_8

Table 8.1 Types of pulmonary infections

Type	Description
Lobar pneumonia	**S. pneumoniae** is the most common etiologic agent. Edema occurs rapidly, with a modest cellular reaction. The consolidation is initially limited to the periphery of the lung, adjacent to the visceral pleura, then the edema progressively diffuses from one acinus to another through Kohn pores. The largest bronchi remain patent, resulting in **air bronchograms** (Fig. 8.1). The lack of volume loss in the consolidated regions is a characteristic feature differentiating an inflammatory process from atelectasis. Sometimes, the exudate can be so massive as to cause an increase in lobe volume, resulting in the **fissure dislocation sign**
Bronchopneumonia	The most common etiologic agents are **S. aureus, Gram-negative bacteria, and some fungi**. Pathologically, bronchopneumonia differs from lobar pneumonia because of the rapid production and diffusion of the exudate, which accumulates in the membranous and respiratory bronchioles. This gives the characteristic bronchiolocentric distribution. Radiologically, it presents with peribronchial cuffing and nodules with indistinct margins. Since the airways are involved, the affected segment or lobe frequently undergoes volume loss. When numerous foci coalesce, bronchopneumonia can be difficult to differentiate from a lobar pneumonia
Lung abscess	**Anaerobic bacteria** are the most common pathogens. The abscess size is variable, ranging from microscopic to lobar extension. It presents as single or multiple cavities, which can be isolated or occurring within a consolidated zone. **Air-fluid levels** are seen in 72% of cases
Interstitial pneumonia	The most common etiologic agents are **viruses and P. jirovecii**. Interstitial pneumonia is characterized by edema and an inflammatory exudate in the septa and peribronchovascular **interstitium**. If associated to bronchiolitis, nodular or linear centrilobular opacities can occur

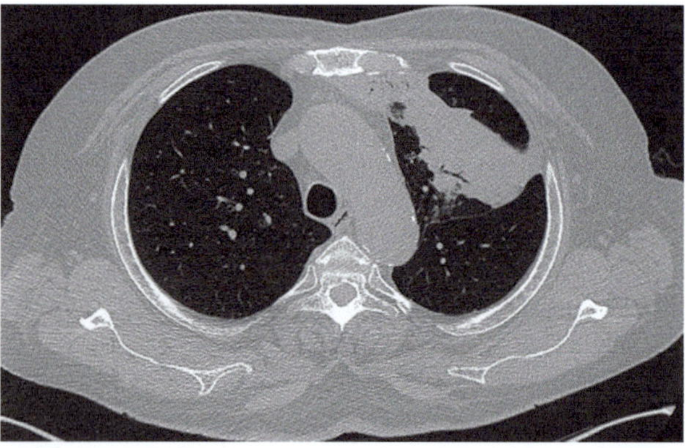

Fig. 8.1 Air bronchogram in lobar pneumonia

the airways; the additional presence of bronchiolar involvement is responsible for centrilobular nodules in a branching pattern (tree-in-bud sign). Abscess formation is not rare (15–30%). Pneumatoceles (thin-walled, air-filled cystic spaces) are common, occurring in 50% of pediatric patients and 15% of adults. They generally develop in the first week and regress spontaneously in weeks or months. The hematogenous staphylococcal pneumonia has a specific radiological presentation characterized by bilateral nodules/masses with poorly defined or confluent margins. It tends to occur in the subpleural area and frequently undergoes cavitation. In about 70% of cases, the nodules develop in the proximity of an artery (feeding vessel sign, Fig. 8.2).

- *Bacteria: Gram-negative cocci*
  - *Klebsiella pneumoniae*: occurs frequently in chronic alcoholics or in patients with comorbidities. It usually presents as a lobar pneumonia, similarly to the pneumococcal one; the main difference is that Klebsiella causes a greater production of inflammatory exudate, which leads to lobar expansion and fissure displacement. In addition, pleural effusions (70%) and abscesses occur more frequently.
  - *Pseudomonas aeruginosa*: the most common and lethal form of HAP. Radiologically, there is bronchopneumonia with bilateral and multifocal consolidations occurring predominantly in the lower lobes. Pleural effusions are common and can rarely lead to empyema.
- *Bacteria: Gram-negative coccobacilli*
  - *Haemophilus influenzae*: responsible for 5–20% of CAPs. Its presentation is extremely heterogeneous: 50% as bronchopneumonia with mono- or bilateral segmental areas of consolidations, 30% as lobar pneumonia, and 20% as interstitial pneumonia. Pleural effusions develop in 50% of cases, cavitations only in 15%.
  - *Legionella spp.*: more common among patients with comorbidities. The typical radiological presentation is a lobar pneumonia rapidly progressing within the same lung or in the contralateral one; this is an important distinguishing feature from pneumococcal pneumonia. Abscesses are common only in immunosuppressed patients.
- *Bacteria: Anaerobes*

  Anaerobic bacteria are responsible for 20–35% of CAPs. The typical radiological pattern is bronchopneumonia with segmental areas of consolidations. If the pneumonia is secondary to aspiration of contaminated materials, a common

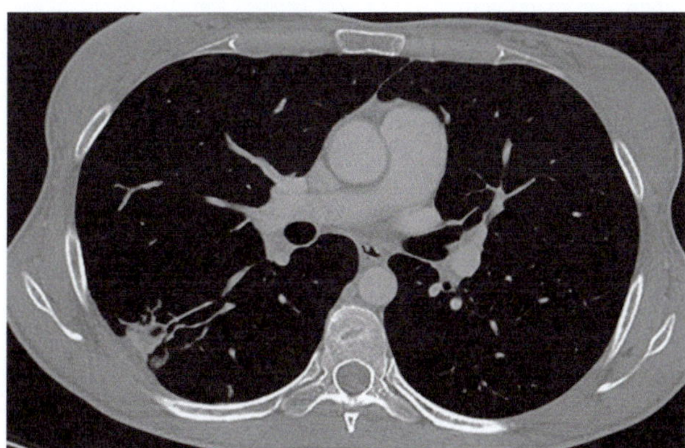

Fig. 8.2 Feeding vessel sign in septic pulmonary embolism. This sign indicates that the lesion has a hematogenous origin; nevertheless, it can also occur in conditions other than septic embolism, e.g., pulmonary infarction, angioinvasive aspergillosis, vasculitis, pulmonary embolism, and AVM

event in intensive care units, the gravity-dependent regions of the lungs are affected, i.e., the posterior segments of the inferior lobes. Cavitations occur in 20–60%.

- *Mycobacteria: Mycobacterium tuberculosis*

  Primary tuberculosis (TB): the initial manifestation is the Ghon focus. In most immunocompetent patients, the primary infection has no radiological manifestations; in some cases, it can become evident as four different patterns:

  - Parenchymal: parenchymal consolidations with the upper lobes more affected than the lower ones.
  - Nodal: hilar lymphadenopathy, often ipsilateral, present in up to 90% of cases of primary TB in the pediatric population. The detection of a peripheral enhancement with low Hounsfield unit values in the central portion of the lymph node is quite characteristic.
  - Airways: when enlarging nodes compress the bronchi atelectasis may occur.
  - Pleural: pleural effusion occurs in 5–10% of children and up to 40% of adults. It is generally associated with the involvement of the lung parenchyma.

  Post-primary tuberculosis: re-activation of the previously acquired infection. Differently from the primary TB it tends to progress, with the extension of the inflammatory foci and necrosis. A typical finding is the initial and prevalent involvement of the apical and posterior segments of the upper lobes. Radiologically, it can present with numerous possible patterns:

  - Air-space consolidation: focal consolidations occur in 50–70% of cases. Usually, it is initially limited to one or more segments of only one lobe; rarely, it involves an entire lobe (tuberculous lobar pneumonia) or can spread via the bronchi to other lobes (tuberculous bronchopneumonia). The presence of hilar lymphadenopathy is less frequent.
  - Cavitations: single or multiple, thin- or thick-walled, with air-fluid levels in 20% of cases (Fig. 8.3). They may disappear after appropriate therapy. A persisting cavitation after therapy is not necessarily an indication of an active status of the disease.

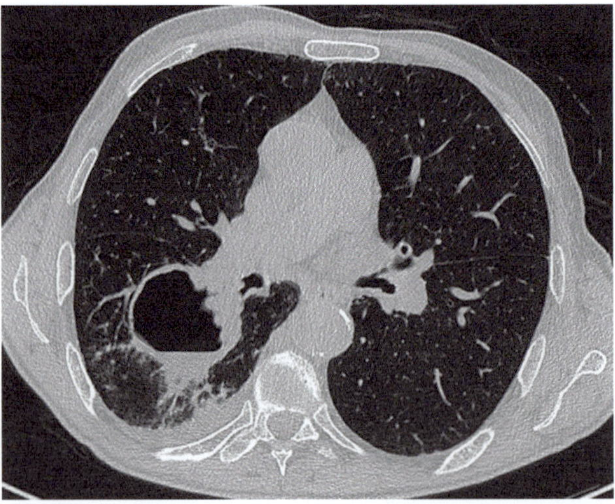

Fig. 8.3 Cavitated tubercular lesion with air-fluid level

- Tuberculoma: roundish opacity more than 1 cm in size, commonly located in the right upper lobe. They are associated to satellite nodules in 80% of cases. They usually remain stable and tend to calcify.
- Focal nodular opacities: 2–10 mm in size, located in two or more segments of the lung and usually associated to consolidated areas. They are distributed in a centrilobular pattern and are often associated to linear opacities that give a tree-in-bud appearance.
- Miliary tuberculosis: well-defined nodules, 1–4 mm in diameter, randomly distributed bilaterally (Fig. 8.4).

• *Atypical Mycobacteria*

As with TB, the radiological pattern of atypical mycobacteria infection can be heterogeneous. Single or multiple cavitations are a common presentation (20–60% of cases). Another pattern is the occurrence of small (<1 cm) bilateral nodular opacities in a patchy and centrilobular distribution. Bronchiectasis and ground-glass opacities are common.

• *Mycoplasma*

Mycoplasma pneumoniae is responsible for 15% of CAPs. The pattern is similar to viral pneumonia, with alveolar-interstitial ground-glass opacities, peribronchial cuffing, and lobar or segmental consolidations. The enlargement of lymph nodes is rare. Pleural effusions are more common (20%) but are unilateral and modest in quantity.

• *Fungi*

- *Histoplasma capsulatum*: both clinical and radiological manifestations are extremely variable. The typical ones are:

  Acute histoplasmosis: poorly defined parenchymal consolidations. Hilar lymphadenopathy, often with calcifications, is common. Bronchiolitis can be associated.

  Histoplasmoma: well-defined nodule of 0.5–3 cm in size, most commonly occurring in lower lobes and sometimes associated to small satellite nodules. They often present central target-like or diffuse calcifications.

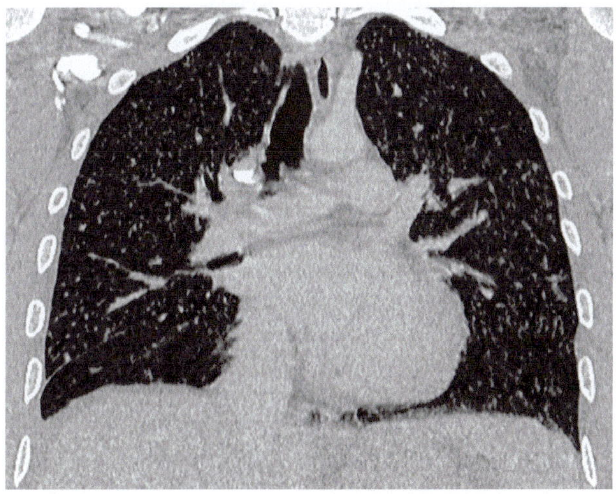

Fig. 8.4 Miliary tuberculosis with millimetric and homogeneous parenchymal nodules, located bilaterally in a random distribution

Chronic pulmonary histoplasmosis: apical segmental consolidations. It can occur after the colonization of bullae with air-fluid levels.

Mediastinal chronic histoplasmosis: hilar or mediastinal masses with calcific components. Bronchovascular obstruction can occur.

- *Pneumocystis jirovecii*: is responsible for a clinically relevant pneumonia in patients with comorbidities, especially AIDS. In the initial phases, the pneumonia presents with a predominantly peri-hilar granular pattern; in the advanced phases, it evolves into air-space consolidations with frequent peripheral reticular/granular pattern. The process is often bilateral, affecting the upper lobes. The typical presentation is bilateral ground-glass opacities in a diffuse or mosaic pattern (Fig. 8.5); in 20–50% of cases, it is associated with interlobular septal thickening. With time, the consolidation can become complete. Enlargement of lymph nodes and pleural effusions are not frequent. A cystic form of the disease with thin-walled cavities is also recognized and may lead to pneumothorax.
- *Aspergillus fumigatus*: Aspergillosis can have three different clinical and radiological presentations (see Table 8.2).

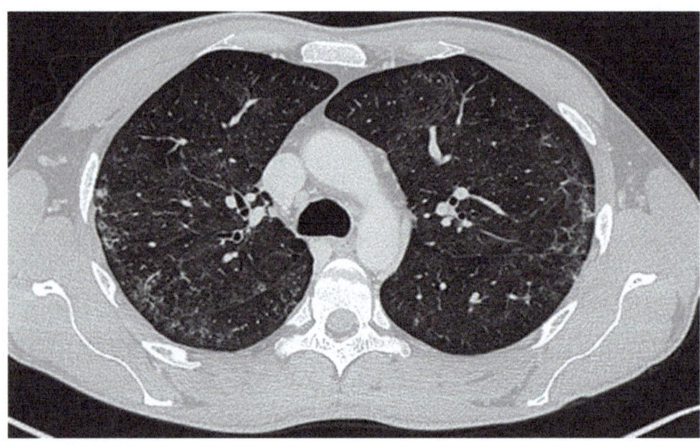

Fig. 8.5 Pneumocystis jirovecii pneumonia, characterized by diffuse ground-glass opacifications

Table 8.2 Aspergillus fumigatus infections

Presentation	Description
Saprophytic aspergillosis: mycetoma	Mass-like collection of fungal hyphae with mucous and cellular debris within a lung cavity (in 25–50% of cases on a pre-existing tuberculosis) or an ectatic bronchus. It is a solid, rounded mass separated from the cavity in which it develops by air (air crescent sign, sometimes not visible if the mass completely fills the cavity). It usually moves after change in patient position
Allergic aspergillosis	Characterized by bronchiectasis and mucoid impactions, or even a mycetoma in case of massive bronchial dilation. Consolidations and atelectasis are less frequent
Invasive aspergillosis	Can have different presentations: • Acute bronchopneumonia: bilateral peribronchial consolidations with poorly defined nodules, 2–5 mm in size, in a centrilobular pattern • Angioinvasive aspergillosis: solid nodule surrounded by a halo of ground-glass opacity (halo sign, Fig. 8.6) caused by hemorrhagic events around necrotic parenchyma. This is a typical sign; nevertheless, it may be present in other neoplastic or infective pathologies. It can progress to frank cavitation

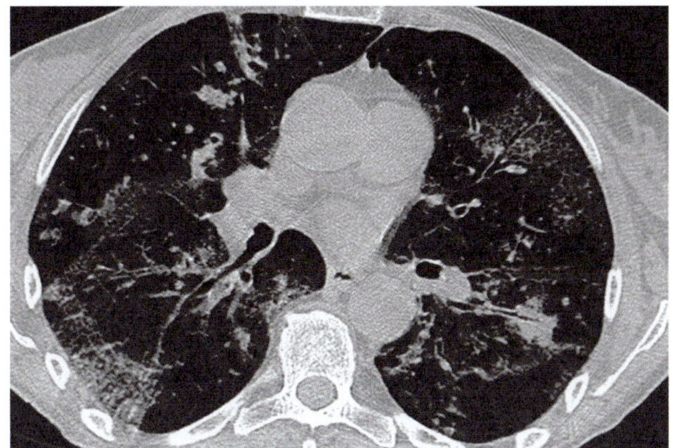

Fig. 8.6 Halo sign in angioinvasive aspergillosis. This pathology presents as pseudo-nodules surrounded by a halo of ground-glass opacity, sign of peripheral hemorrhagic events. In this figure, there are also bilateral ground-glass opacifications

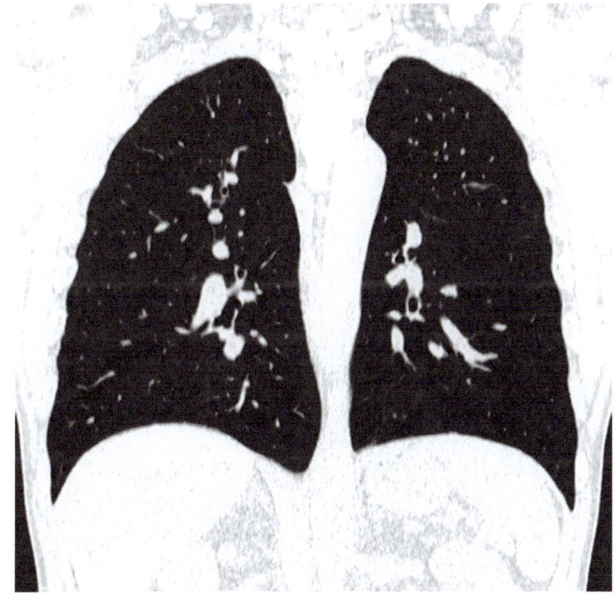

Fig. 8.7 Atypical pneumonia of viral etiology, presenting with multiple and bilateral ground-glass opacities

- *Viruses*
  - *Cytomegalovirus*: a common etiologic agent in immunosuppressed patients (AIDS or post-transplant), occurring only rarely in immunocompetent subjects. The typical presentation is ground-glass opacities, parenchymal consolidations, and bilateral reticulonodular opacities (Fig. 8.7).
  - *Varicella virus*: occurs as nodular opacities 5–10 mm in size, generally in the peripheral zone but tend to coalesce in peri-hilar location. They can evolve into consolidations. Rarely, it presents as diffuse calcific foci in both lungs.

Bronchiolitis

Numerous lung pathologies can cause an inflammation of the membranous and respiratory bronchioles and therefore the radiological manifestation of bronchiolitis is extremely variable. The thickening of the bronchiolar walls or the filling of their lumens results in the characteristic centrilobular nodules and linear opacities (tree-in-bud appearance, Fig. 8.8). This presentation is common in acute infectious bronchiolitis and can be associated to alveolar-interstitial opacities.

The narrowing of the bronchiolar lumens causes a reduction in ventilation with consequent reflex vasoconstriction redistributing the blood flow in the lung parenchyma. This causes areas with different attenuations that appear as a mosaic pattern (mosaic perfusion). Differently, a mono- or bilateral parenchymal consolidation is typical of the Bronchiolitis Obliterans Organizing Pneumonia (BOOP). Ground-glass opacities are also common in both respiratory bronchiolitis and BOOP. Table 8.3 summarizes the different types of bronchiolitis and their typical anatomopathological and radiological presentation.

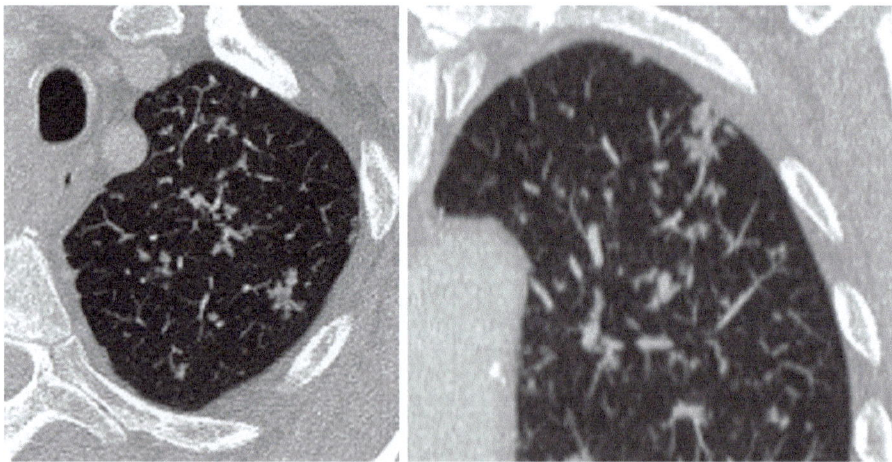

Fig. 8.8 Tree-in-bud appearance, representing multiple centrilobular nodules associated to linear opacities

Table 8.3 Classification of bronchiolitis

Classification	Description
Acute bronchiolitis	Acute bronchiolar inflammation associated to a variable degree of inflammation in the adjacent parenchyma. It presents as linear branching nodular opacities in a diffuse or patchy pattern
Chronic bronchiolitis	Chronic inflammation and fibrosis. It is the typical histological finding in chronic smokers. Radiologically, it presents with centrilobular nodules
Respiratory bronchiolitis	Accumulation of macrophages within bronchioles with lymphocytic infiltration and fibrosis. It is the first pathological alteration in smokers. It presents as ground-glass and ill-defined centrilobular opacities, located mainly in the superior lobes
Bronchiolitis obliterans organizing pneumonia (BOOP)	Bronchiolar fibrosis with lumen stenosis. It can progress to bronchiolar necrosis with occlusion of the airway lumen. In the lung parenchyma, there are initial alterations in the ventilation-perfusion ratio in a mosaic pattern, with consequent formation of consolidations and ground-glass opacities

Suggested Readings

Al-Ghanem S, et al. Bronchiolitis obliterans organizing pneumonia: pathogenesis, clinical features, imaging and therapy review. Ann Thorac Med. 2008;3(2):67–75.

Franquet T, et al. Imaging of pulmonary viral pneumonia. Radiology. 2011;260(1):18–39.

Kim EA, et al. Viral pneumonias in adults: radiologic and pathologic findings. Radiographics. 2002;22:S137–49.

Presentation and Diagnosis of Interstitial Lung Diseases

9

Alessandro Maria Ferrazza and Paolo Baldassarri

Diffuse interstitial lung disease is a heterogeneous group of lung pathologies with similar clinical presentations. Radiologists and pathologists attempted to identify precise diagnostic criteria. Often, the pattern and distribution of the disease allow to narrow down the possible diagnoses, but the correlation with the clinical presentation is essential.

The main radiological patterns are:

- Nodular
- Septal
- Cystic
- Alveolar (ground-glass)
- Reticular
- Honeycombing

To recognize the radiological pattern of the disease, it is necessary to search and study on HRCT images the secondary pulmonary lobule (SPL) that is the smallest structural unit in the lung. It is a roughly polyhedral structure, 1–2 cm in size, lined by connective tissue septa; the lobules in the peripheral regions of the lung are larger and more regular in shape, becoming smaller and more irregular in the central portions. Each SPL is constituted by 3–15 acini and 30–50 alveoli and is fed by a small lobular bronchiole and a pulmonary artery branch. These structures run in parallel in the central portion of the lobule and are therefore described as centrilobular. In the peripheral region, the venous and lymphatic vessels are contained in the interlobular interstitium.

A. M. Ferrazza (✉) · P. Baldassarri
Department of Radiological, Oncological and Pathological Sciences, Sapienza University of Rome, Rome, Italy

I. Carbone, M. Anzidei (eds.), *Thoracic Radiology*,
https://doi.org/10.1007/978-3-030-35765-8_9

The SPL is composed by three main elements:

- *The interlobular septa:* normally about 0.1 mm thick and therefore not visible on HRCT except in the peripheral region where they are slightly thicker and can barely be identified. The venous branches running within them have a caliber of about 0.5 mm and can, therefore, be visualized. Diseases affecting the venous or lymphatic systems of the lung will affect this region, e.g., "perilobular" patterns.
- *The centrilobular structures:* consist of the intralobular arterial and bronchial branches. In normal conditions, it is possible to identify the lobular artery (1 mm), the terminal artery (0.7 mm), and the acinar artery (0.5 mm). The bronchial branches contain air and cannot be visualized as their wall thickness is inferior to the lower limit of resolution on HRCT (0.15 mm). When the bronchiolar lumens become plugged with dense materials such as fluids, blood, or pus, the tracings of the intralobular branches become visible on HRCT as branched structures terminating in small nodules (tree-in-bud appearance).
- *The lobular parenchyma and acini:* not visible on HRCT under normal conditions. They include the functional units of the lung, i.e., the alveoli and the capillary bed with their supportive structures of connective tissue (intralobular interstitium). In some pathologies, e.g., inflammatory diseases, the involvement of the acinus appears as a small intralobular nodular opacity, about 0.6–1 mm in size.

Nodular Pattern

The nodular pattern is characterized by nodules less than 1 cm in size with variable characteristics and distribution, based on which it can subdivided into:

- Nodules in a random pattern (Fig. 9.1)
- Nodules in a miliary pattern (Figs. 9.1 and 9.2)
- Nodules in a centrilobular (or bronchovascular) pattern (Fig. 9.3)
- Nodules in a lymphatic or perilymphatic pattern (Fig. 9.4)

Nodules in a Random Pattern

They are usually secondary to pathologies with hematogenous dissemination (Table 9.1). Thus, they are:

- Diffuse (and never focal, as can occur in the bronchovascular pattern)
- More numerous in the periphery (within 2–3 cm from the pleura) and at the bases (where there is more blood flow)

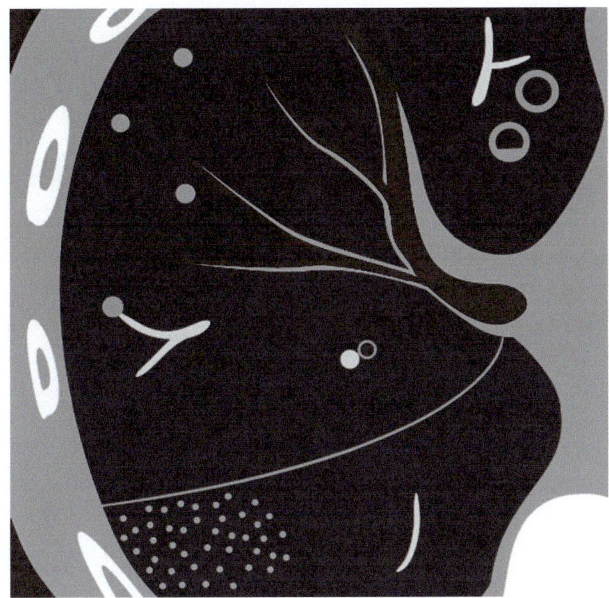

Fig. 9.1 Nodules in a random pattern

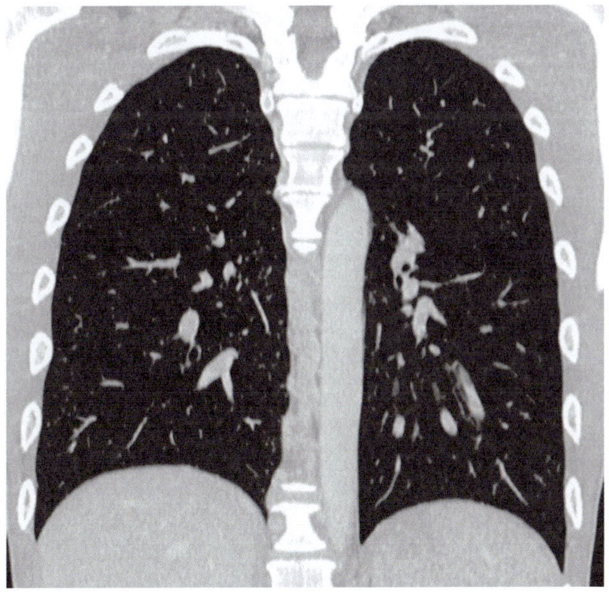

Fig. 9.2 Patient with miliary dissemination of tuberculosis

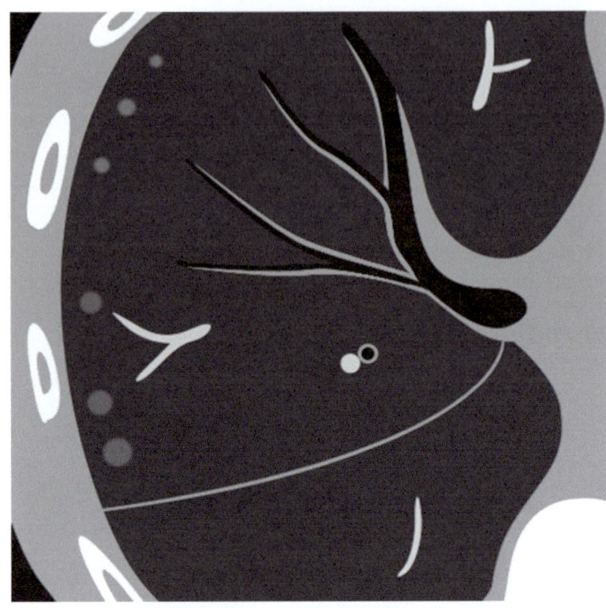

Fig. 9.3 Nodules in a centrilobular pattern

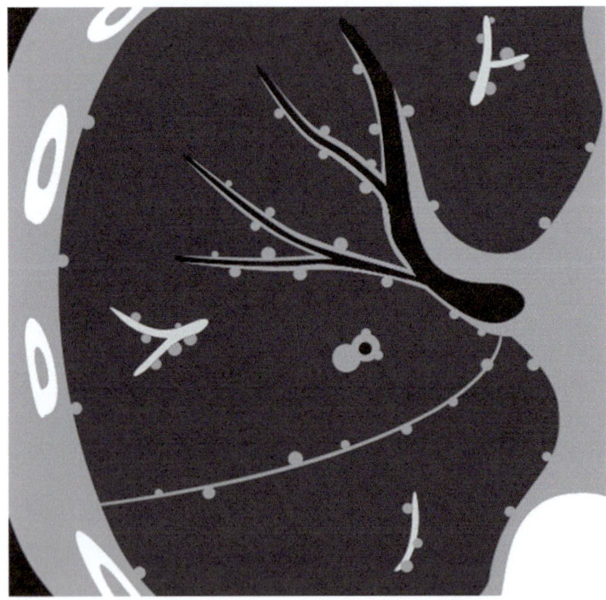

Fig. 9.4 Nodules in a lymphatic or perilymphatic pattern

Table 9.1 Differential diagnosis of nodules in a random pattern

Common	
Hematogenous metastases	Nodules of variable shape and size. The most common primary cancers are gastrointestinal, pulmonary, mammary or melanoma and sarcoma Calcified hematogenous metastases are most commonly secondary to chondrosarcoma and osteosarcoma or, especially when treated with chemotherapy, colon and ovarian cancer A halo of ground-glass attenuation can be appreciated if perilesional hemorrhage occurs Miliary metastases present as numerous nodules of the same size and are typically secondary to medullary thyroid, renal, head and neck, ovarian and testicular cancer and melanoma
Miliary infections	Mycobacterial, histoplasmosis, or viral infections
Septic emboli	Fever is associated. Cavitation usually occurs within 24 h (Fig. 9.1, upper part). It mostly occurs in patients with central lines, right-sided endocarditis, or in intravenous drug abusers
Intravascular talcosis	High-density pinpoint nodules due to the intravenous use of drugs mixed with talc
Less common	
Vasculitis	Nodules are due to hemosiderin-laden macrophages that accumulate after localized hemorrhages. On CT, they are seen as ground-glass opacities, in general with a centrilobular distribution

- Possibly associated to a feeding vessel, that is, an arterial vessel entering the nodule (Fig. 9.1, in the center)

If they are few in number, it may be difficult to distinguish this pattern from a centrilobular or perilymphatic one.

Nodules in a Miliary Pattern

They are secondary to pathologies with hematogenous dissemination (Tables 9.2 and 9.3) and have the following characteristics:

- Small nodules (<5 mm), too many to be counted (Fig. 9.1, lower part; Fig. 9.2);
- Random distribution within the SPL.

CXR may be negative due to their small size.

Dense or calcific nodules in a miliary pattern can be secondary to healed histoplasmosis, healed chickenpox, thyroid metastases after radioactive Iodine-131 treatment, talcosis, and pulmonary alveolar microlithiasis.

Table 9.2 Differential diagnosis of nodules in a miliary pattern

Common	
Primary or post-primary tuberculosis	Occurring mainly in immunocompromised patients. The sputum smear is usually negative, often needing a transbronchial biopsy for diagnosis
Atypical mycobacterial diseases	Nodules are often centrilobular but can occasionally be in a miliary pattern
Viral infections	Usually influenza and cytomegalovirus
Chickenpox and histoplasmosis	After healing, miliary calcified nodules may occur
Fungal infections	Can be observed when the infection disseminates in immunocompromised patients
Blastomycosis	Similar to tuberculosis
Metastases	Secondary to medullary thyroid, renal, head and neck, ovarian and testicular cancer, and melanoma
Less common	
Talcosis	Secondary to intravenous drug abuse
Pulmonary alveolar microlithiasis	Calcific nodules with subpleural sparing of the lung (black pleura sign)
Sarcoidosis and silicosis	Usually perilymphatic nodules but they can appear as miliary
Langerhans cell histiocytosis	Usually centrilobular nodules but they can appear as miliary
Hypersensitivity pneumonitis	
Bronchioloalveolar carcinoma	Ground-glass nodules, usually centrilobular, but in case of hematogenous dissemination they can be miliary and random

Table 9.3 Differential diagnosis between mycobacterial miliary nodules and metastases

	Mycobacterial nodules	Metastatic nodules
Appearance	<5 mm	Bigger and well-defined
Background ground-glass	Common	Rare
Location	Superior lobes	Inferior lobes

Nodules in a Centrilobular Pattern

These nodules are located in the bronchovascular core of the SPL and are a typical manifestation of bronchiolocentric or bronchiolar interstitial lung diseases (Table 9.4). They are:

- Located at least 5–10 mm from the pleural surface or the interlobar fissures or the SPL margins
- Generally of ground-glass density
- Associated to other signs of bronchiolar obstruction:
  - Tree-in-bud opacities: the bronchioles are dilated and plugged by dense contents (mucus, pus, or fluid) and peribronchial inflammation is present
  - Mosaic pattern: due to hyperinflation of some SPLs
- Common in bronchiectasis of any cause

Table 9.4 Differential diagnosis of nodules in a centrilobular pattern

Common	
Infectious bronchiolitis	Secondary to bacterial, viral, fungal, or mycobacterial infections; typical of tuberculosis with endobronchial spread
Respiratory bronchiolitis	Correlated to smoking (at least 2 years of smoking history) and characterized by pigmented macrophages within the respiratory bronchioles. There are centrilobular nodules with prevalent involvement of the superior lobes and progression to emphysema
Subacute hypersensitivity pneumonitis	Formation of granulomas in response to various types of antigens (farmer's lung or bird fancier's lung). There are centrilobular nodules that progress to thin-walled cysts and a prevalent involvement of the upper lobes with sparing of the inferior zones and costophrenic angles (typical aspect). A mosaic pattern can co-occur
Langerhans cell histiocytosis	Correlated to smoking, it is most likely due to an allergic response to some smoke components. Centrilobular nodules evolve into thin-walled cysts that can aggregate in bizarre shapes. There is prevalent involvement of the upper lobes and sparing of the inferior zones and costophrenic angles
Follicular bronchiolitis	Associated to hyperplasia of the Bronchus-Associated Lymphoid Tissue (BALT) in pathologies such as rheumatoid arthritis, Sjögren's, AIDS, infections, and hypersensitivity reactions. There are centrilobular nodules, subpleural nodules, thin-walled cysts, and ground-glass areas. It can be associated to interlobular septal thickening
Less common	
Aspiration	Usually secondary to chronic leguminous material aspiration. Characterized by centrilobular nodules in a gravity-dependent pattern
Bronchioloalveolar carcinoma	Early on, it can appear as centrilobular nodules
Vasculitis	Centrilobular nodules with ground-glass opacity due to the presence of hemosiderin-laden macrophages after localized hemorrhages
Pulmonary hypertension	Centrilobular nodules can be present in all forms of pulmonary hypertension. They are due to plexogenic arteriopathy in primary pulmonary arterial hypertension, to capillary dilatations in pulmonary veno-occlusive disease, and to capillary proliferation in pulmonary capillary hemangiomatosis
Kidney failure	Calcific nodules (calcified-cauliflower sign) can be seen in the most advanced stages of kidney failure
Laryngeal papillomatosis	Nodules can be seen in 1% of cases and are due to endobronchial seeding in the lung. The centrilobular nodules tend to cavitate forming cysts

Nodules in a Lymphatic or Perilymphatic Pattern

These are nodules located around the lymphatic vessels and the perilymphatic channels (Figs. 9.4 and 9.5; Table 9.5). Their characteristics are as follows:

- Well-defined nodules (2–5 mm)
- Axial distribution: in the peribronchovascular interstitium, from the hilum to the periphery

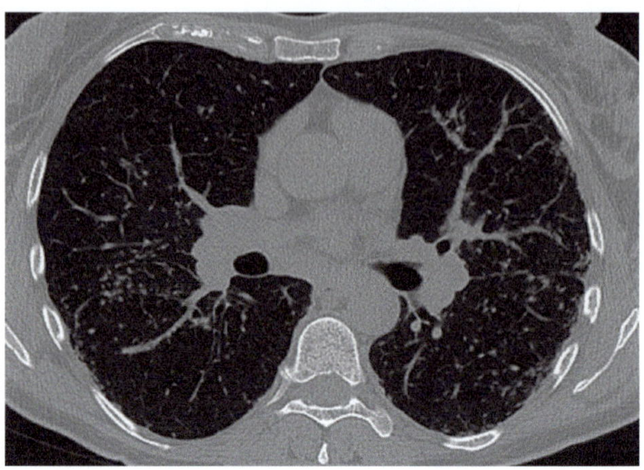

Fig. 9.5 Nodules in a perilymphatic pattern in a patient with sarcoidosis

Table 9.5 Differential diagnosis of nodules in a perilymphatic pattern

Common	
Sarcoidosis	Perilymphatic nodules in an axial distribution from the hilum, with hilar and mediastinal adenopathy. They can aggregate forming masses (alveolar sarcoids) which can contain calcifications, i.e., the typical galaxy sign, characterized by a central mass surrounded by small nodules. It progresses to fibrosis with a reticular pattern
Berylliosis	Same presentation as sarcoidosis but with a history of occupational exposure to beryllium
Round-shaped particles inhalation	Perilymphatic nodules in an axial distribution from the hilum, with hilar lymphadenopathy. They can aggregate forming masses in the dorsal regions. It progresses to fibrosis. It is more prevalent in the superior lobes, being more ventilated. The most typical forms are silicosis, coal worker's pneumoconiosis (typical hilar eggshell calcifications in 5% of cases), talcosis, and siderosis
Lymphangitic carcinomatosis	Perilymphatic nodules in a predominantly axial distribution (75%). Usually associated to adenocarcinoma. It differs from pneumoconiosis in that whole lobes or a whole lung are usually spared, the lung architecture is preserved (while it is distorted in sarcoidosis and silicosis), and pleural effusions can be present (never present in pneumoconiosis)
Less common	
Lymphocytic Interstitial Pneumonia (LIP)	Idiopathic or secondary to HIV infection, EBV infection, dysproteinemia, or Sjögren's syndrome. It appears as nodules in a perilymphatic pattern, thin-walled cysts (80% of cases), and ground-glass opacities (100% of cases)
Lymphoma	Non-Hodgkin (25% of cases) or Hodgkin (40% of cases) with lung involvement. Pulmonary nodules >1 cm in size, often with bronchogram
Miliary infections	CMV, tuberculous, or fungal infections. It appears as pulmonary micronodules, usually in a random or miliary pattern, but they can mimic a perilymphatic pattern
Follicular bronchiolitis	Nodules are more often in a centrilobular pattern, associated to subpleural nodules, thin-walled cysts, ground-glass areas, and interlobular septal thickening. It can mimic a perilymphatic pattern
Kaposi sarcoma	Occurs in AIDS-affected patients. Ill-defined nodules in a predominantly perihilar distribution
Amyloidosis	May present as perilymphatic nodules in a peripheral (subpleural) distribution, with nodular thickening of the peribronchovascular structures and septal thickening

HIV human immunodeficiency virus, *EBV* Epstein–Barr virus, *CMV* Cytomegalovirus

- Peripheral distribution: in the subpleural interstitium, in the interstitium of fissures and SPL contour
- Associated to involvement of mediastinal lymph nodes

Some diseases can start as a bronchovascular pattern (through inhalation) and then progress to a lymphatic pattern (through dissemination).

Differential Diagnosis of Nodular Patterns

The distinction of the nodular patterns depends mostly on the location, pattern, and appearance of the nodules (Table 9.6). The presence of accessory signs of airways obstruction, such as a mosaic pattern or tree-in-bud opacities, can help to distinguish the centrilobular pattern from the others, in which they rarely occur.

- *Tree-in-bud opacities (TIB):* They appear as quite defined centrilobular nodules (2–4 mm) from which linear opacities spread out in three or four V-shaped or Y-shaped branches (Fig. 9.6). They correlate to bronchiolar pathologies and are

Table 9.6 Differences between nodular patterns

	Random	Centrilobular	Perilymphatic
Etiology	Hematogenous	Aerogenous	Lymphogenous
Location	Inferior lobes (more blood flow)	Superior lobes (more ventilation)	Variable
Pattern	Random	In the center of SPL	Axial or peripheral perilymphatic
Appearance of nodules	Variable—a feeding vessel may be present	Ground-glass is suggestive	Denser and more well-defined
Signs of airways obstruction	Absent	Present	Absent

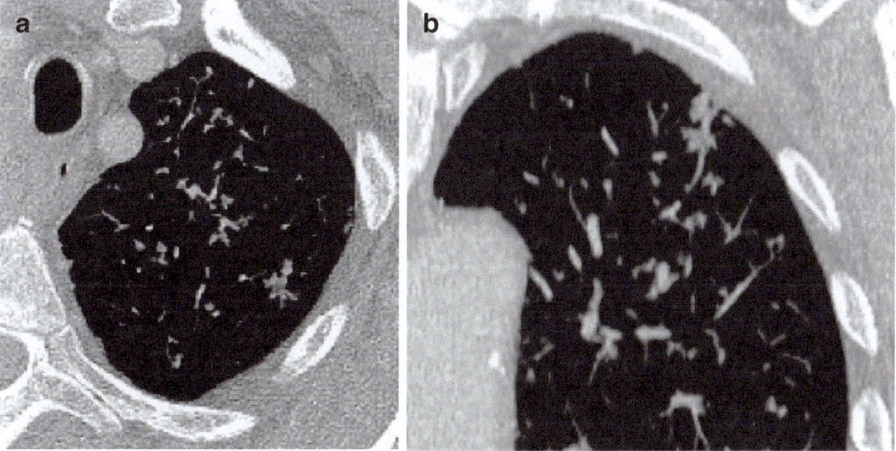

Fig. 9.6 Tree-in-bud opacities in a patient with tuberculosis: (**a**) axial view, (**b**) coronal view

caused by the dilation of the bronchiolar lumen, filled with mucus, pus, or fluid, and to the thickening of their walls. Rarely, they can be secondary to pathologies with hematogenous dissemination such as metastatic tumors or intravenous drug abuse, which can cause arteriolar dilation (Table 9.7).

- *Mosaic pattern:* There are areas of attenuation corresponding to the SPL (Fig. 9.7; Tables 9.8 and 9.9). It can be caused by:

Table 9.7 Differential diagnosis of tree-in-bud opacities (TIB)

Possible diagnoses when airways are normal	
Infectious bronchiolitis	Most frequent cause of TIB pattern. The bronchoalveolar lavage, performed when the cause is not immediately evident, is frequently positive for germs. The most frequent etiologies are: • Mycobacterium tuberculosis or atypical mycobacteria • Mycoplasma pneumoniae • Viral pneumonia, influenza • Other bacterial, viral, fungal etiologies • Diffuse panbronchiolitis: unknown etiology, can cause respiratory failure
Aspiration	TIB pattern in gravity-dependent regions: • Exogenous aspiration: in case of unconscious patients, alcoholism, swallowing disorders (posterior and basal lung segments in supine and standing patients, respectively) • Endogenous aspiration: aspiration of the contents in the M. tuberculosis cavitations (from apical cavitations to basal segments or contralateral lung)
Rare bronchial causes	Other rare causes of TIB with normal airways are: • Follicular bronchiolitis: typical centrilobular nodular pattern • Primary pulmonary lymphoma: similar to follicular bronchiolitis • Bronchioloalveolar carcinoma: typical presentation with ground-glass opacity and bronchogram • Asthma: late finding in severe asthmatic crisis
Vascular causes	Rare causes, characterized by absence of air-trapping and presence of enlarged pulmonary arteries: • Intravascular metastases from angiosarcoma, renal carcinoma, hepatic carcinoma; a characteristic finding is the 90° angle of the branches in the TIB pattern • Intravenous drug abuse: granulomatous reaction to injected substances
Possible diagnoses when bronchiectasis and proximal bronchial wall thickening are present (TIB pattern is seen in 25% of patients with bronchiectasis)	
Infectious bronchiolitis	Usually when secondary to M. avium complex. Prevalently located in the middle lobe and lingula
Cystic fibrosis, primary ciliary dyskinesia	Located in the superior lobes
Allergic bronchopulmonary aspergillosis	Located in the superior lobes
Common variable immunodeficiency	Secondary to recurrent bronchial infections

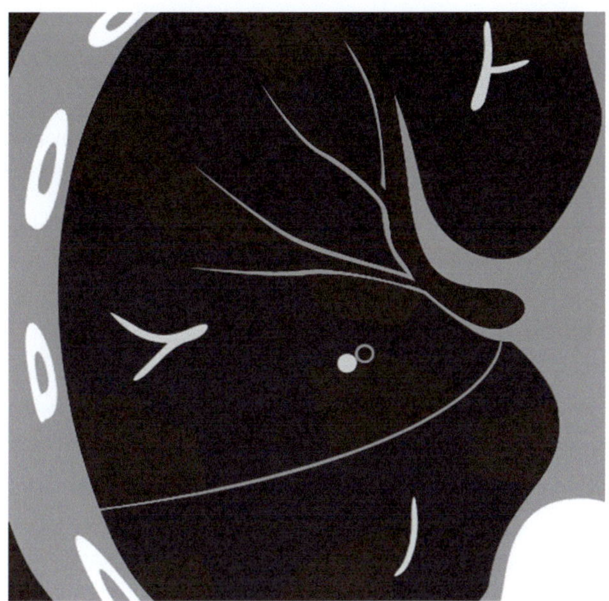

Fig. 9.7 Mosaic pattern

Table 9.8 Differences between mosaic patterns of different etiologies

	Bronchial	Vascular	Patchy ground-glass
Symptoms	Dyspnea, cough, wheezing	Dyspnea, no cough, or wheezing	Dyspnea, possible cough or wheezing
Pulmonary function tests	Obstructive pattern, DLCO normal	Normal pattern, DLCO significantly reduced	Restrictive pattern, DLCO variable
Caliber of vessels in regions with less attenuation (difficult to appreciate)	Reduced	Reduced	Normal
Air-trapping on CT during expiration	Prominent	None (except in acute pulmonary embolism due to reflex bronchoconstriction)	None

- Obstruction of the small airways: emphysematous areas due to air-trapping
- Vascular occlusive diseases: less vascularized areas. Usually, bronchoconstriction with air-trapping is also present in these regions as the lung attempts to maintain the ventilation-perfusion ratio within normal values
- Patchy lung diseases: ground-glass opacification of only some SPL
- Mixed: interstitial and small-airways disease

It can be observed in 60% of normal subjects during expiration (maximum 1 lobule per CT section, mainly in the superior and ventral lobes).

It can be difficult to recognize if almost all lobules are hyperextended.

Table 9.9 Differential diagnosis of mosaic pattern

Bronchogenic forms	
Bronchiolitis obliterans	A mosaic pattern is observed in 50% of cases. It can be cryptogenic, post-infectious (usually viral), toxic (from inhalation of fumes as in Silo-Filler's disease or from penicillamine), secondary to bone marrow and lung transplant (50% of cases), or to rheumatoid arthritis and chronic inflammatory bowel diseases
Acute/subacute hypersensitivity pneumonitis	Formation of granulomas in response to various types of antigens (farmer's lung or bird fancier's lung, hot tub lung). It is characterized by: • Centrilobular nodules of ground-glass density which evolve into thin-walled cysts (1–14 cysts) • Mosaic pattern, present in 85% of cases • Prevalent involvement of superior lobes and sparing of inferior zones and costophrenic angles (typical aspect)
Infectious bronchiolitis (viral)	Usually in viral forms. The typical aspect is the presence of centrilobular nodules, but a mosaic pattern can be associated
Normal aging-related changes in the lung	A mosaic pattern may be observed in 25% of older patients and is not correlated to smoking habits
Cystic fibrosis	Usually associated to bronchiectasis
False mosaic pattern	Artifact that can be observed when the lung window setting is too narrow
Bronchial asthma	A mosaic pattern is rare. It occurs in 3% of cases, especially in severe asthma
Panlobular emphysema	More commonly there are only regions with less attenuation; a mosaic pattern can be observed in the inferior lobes
Arterial forms	
Pulmonary arterial hypertension	• From vascular causes (75%): chronic thromboembolism, vasculitis, primary pulmonary hypertension, pulmonary veno-occlusive disease (PVOD), pulmonary capillary hemangiomatosis (PCH). In particular, the post-capillary forms (PVOD and PCH) have additional features: – Interlobular septal thickening – Pleural effusion – Mediastinal adenopathy • From cardiac causes (10%) • From pulmonary causes (5%)

Septal Pattern

It represents the interlobular septal thickening of the SPL and is seen as short lines in the periphery of the lung that arrive to the pleura. They can have different morphology: smooth, nodular, irregular.

The most common diagnoses are (Tables 9.10 and 9.11):

- Pulmonary edema: smooth (Figs. 9.8a and 9.9)
- Pulmonary fibrosis: irregular
- Lymphangitic carcinomatosis: smooth or nodular (Fig. 9.8b). It can be associated with the following:
  - Prevalently septal pattern with nodular and irregular thickening
  - Often entire lobes or the contralateral lung are spared
  - Hilar lymphadenopathy

Table 9.10 Differential diagnosis of septal pattern (acute forms)

Common	
Cardiogenic pulmonary edema	Prevalent involvement of gravity-dependent regions and association to effusion. The prevalence of crazy paving pattern is 10–20%
Pneumocystis pneumonia	Prevalent involvement of perihilar regions and superior lobes. It is associated to pneumatoceles (observed only in HIV patients)
Acute Interstitial Pneumonia (AIP), Acute Respiratory Distress Syndrome (ARDS), and Diffuse Alveolar Damage (DAD)	Cause of acute respiratory failure requiring mechanical ventilation (DAD is the histological presentation of AIP and ARDS). The radiological presentation is characterized prevalently by ground-glass opacities, but also crazy paving can be observed (30–66%)
Less common	
Diffuse alveolar hemorrhage	Characterized by different phases: • Hemorrhage in alveolar spaces resulting in consolidations or ground-glass • Removal of blood by macrophages, which migrate in the interstitium and in the septa (2–3 days), with crazy paving pattern (10–20%) • Removal of macrophages by the lymphatic system (7–14 days)
Acute eosinophilic pneumonia	Characterized by migrating ground-glass areas, less frequently by crazy paving (10–20%)

Table 9.11 Differential diagnosis of septal pattern (subacute and chronic forms)

Common	
Pulmonary Alveolar Proteinosis (PAP)	Diffuse crazy paving pattern. The clinical symptoms (cough and dyspnea) are typically less severe than the radiological presentation
Less common	
Non-Specific Interstitial Pneumonia (NSIP)	Idiopathic or secondary to scleroderma, rheumatoid arthritis, drug-induced lung disease It is characterized prevalently by ground-glass, reticular pattern, and traction bronchiectasis. There can also be a septal thickening more evident at the bases and at the periphery of the lung. Subpleural sparing of the lung in the dorsal regions is characteristic
Cryptogenic Organizing Pneumonia (COP)	Pathology characterized by granulomatous polypoid structures growing inside the bronchi. Different patterns can be observed: • Subpleural and peribronchial consolidations or ground-glass opacities (90%) with air bronchogram of variable shape and dimension (ranging from few centimeters to entire lobes), in a migrating pattern • Perilobular pattern: opacities or ground-glass at the periphery of the SPL that can mimic a septal pattern • Multiple or single opacities with the reversed halo sign, i.e., central ground-glass surrounded by consolidation, at least 2 mm • Ground-glass in peripheral zones, more common than crazy paving (10–20%)
Chronic eosinophilic pneumonia	The most frequent presentation is ground-glass opacity, but it can present as crazy paving in peripheral zones (10–20%)
Lymphangitic carcinomatosis	In general, it involves one or more lobes asymmetrically

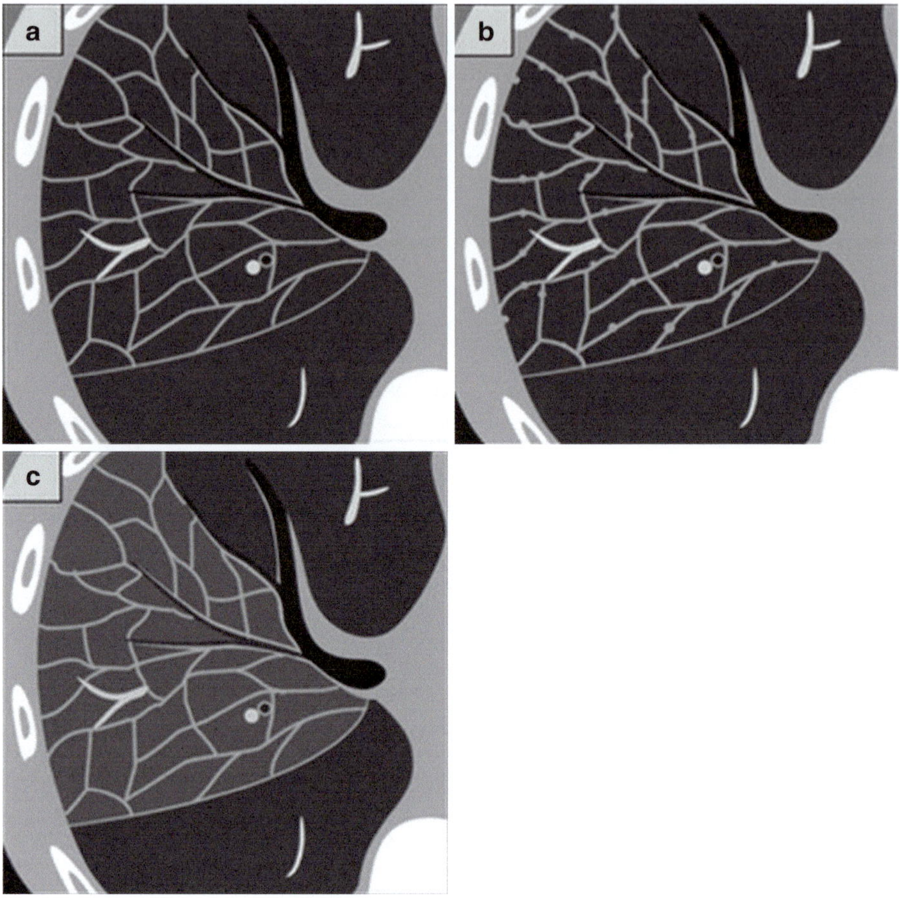

Fig. 9.8 Septal pattern: (**a**) Smooth septal thickening, (**b**) Nodular septal thickening, (**c**) Ground-glass with superimposed septal thickening, also called "crazy paving" pattern

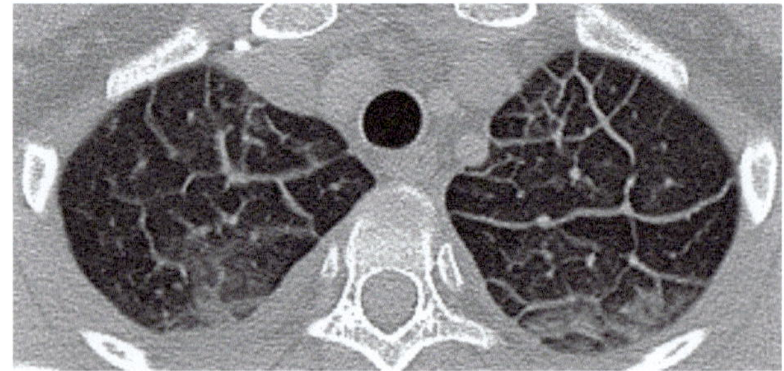

Fig. 9.9 Septal pattern with smooth septal thickening in a patient with non-cardiogenic pulmonary edema secondary to CHT

The septal pattern can be associated with ground-glass opacities, leading to the so-called crazy paving pattern (Fig. 9.8c). This was initially described in pulmonary alveolar proteinosis, where the ground-glass appearance is due to the partial alveolar filling with proteinaceous material, and the septal pattern is due to the thickening of the SPL's septa or the accumulation of material at the periphery of the air spaces.

Cystic Pattern

It is characterized by air-filled or fluid-filled spaces with more or less defined walls. Superior lobes are more involved because the apical regions of the lung are subjected to greater gravity-induced stretching. All diseases causing a cystic pattern increase the risk of pneumothorax (Table 9.12).

Initially, pulmonary function tests show a restrictive pattern with reduction of lung diffusion for CO; later, they present an obstructive pattern.

Table 9.12 Differential diagnosis of cystic pattern

Common	
Pulmonary emphysema	Permanent enlargement of the distal air spaces up to the terminal bronchioles secondary to smoke, α1AT deficiency, intravenous drug abuse. It can be centrilobular, paraseptal, or panlobular
Langerhans cell histiocytosis	Centrilobular nodules that evolve into thin-walled cysts, which can aggregate in bizarre shapes. They spare the inferior zones and costophrenic angles. It correlates with smoke exposure and most likely is an allergic response to some smoke components (Fig. 9.10, on the left)
Pneumatoceles	Thin-walled transient cysts that usually resolve within months. The main causes are: • Staphylococcal pneumonia • Pneumocystis jirovecii pneumonia in AIDS-affected patients (30%) • Trauma
Less common	
Lymphangioleiomyomatosis (LAM)	Observed only in women. On CT, there are uniform cysts throughout the lung which slowly replace the parenchyma (Fig. 9.10, on the right). Possible complications are pneumothorax and chylothorax
Subacute hypersensitivity pneumonitis	Characterized by centrilobular nodules evolving into thin-walled cysts; usually 1–14 cysts are observed in 10% of cases
Lymphocytic Interstitial Pneumonia (LIP)	Can be idiopathic or secondary to infections (HIV, EBV), dysproteinemia, and Sjögren's syndrome. On CT, there are thin-walled cysts in 80% of cases, usually less than 20 in number, ground-glass appearance (100%), and nodules in a perilymphatic pattern
Desquamative Interstitial Pneumonia (DIP)	The etiology is unknown; it has a higher prevalence in heavy smokers. It is characterized by thin-walled cysts (80%) of usually small dimension in the lower lobes and ground-glass opacities
Idiopathic Pulmonary Fibrosis (IPF)	Presents with basal or peripheral honeycombing (multiple rows of cysts, 0.3–1 cm in dimension). It can mimic a cystic pattern
Laryngeal papillomatosis	Characterized by centrilobular nodules affecting gravity-dependent regions; they can evolve into cysts
Coccidioidomycosis	Fungal infection that is endemic in the southwestern regions of the USA (valley fever). In its late form, it presents as often single, thin-walled cysts in the superior lobes

α1AT Alpha-1 antitrypsin, *HIV* human immunodeficiency virus, *EBV* Epstein–Barr virus

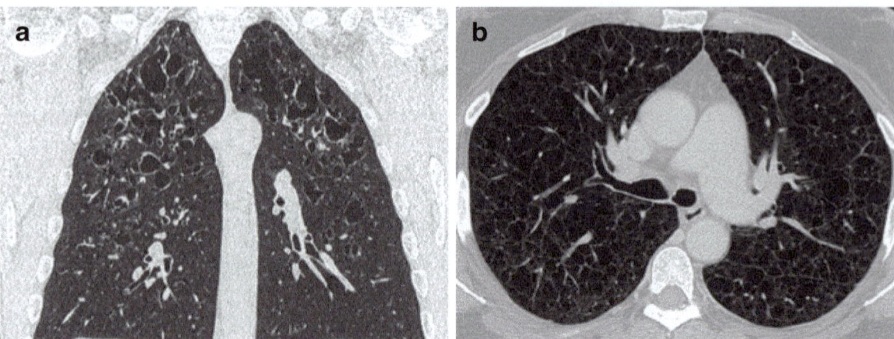

Fig. 9.10 Cystic pattern: (**a**) Langerhans cell granulomatosis. Characteristically dysmorphic thin-walled cysts. (**b**) Lymphangioleiomyomatosis

Alveolar Pattern: Ground-Glass Opacities

The alveolar patterns are ground-glass opacity and parenchymal consolidation.

The ground-glass opacities are characterized by an increased opacity of the lung parenchyma that does not obscure the underlying structures (Fig. 9.11). In the pulmonary consolidation, the bronchovascular structures are obscured.

Ground-glass opacities represent an acute process or an acute flare of a chronic disease (Table 9.13). The radiological presentation is due to:

- Partial filling of air spaces (edema, hemorrhage, pus)
- Interstitial thickening secondary to edema, inflammation, or fibrosis, usually associated to a reticular pattern or traction bronchiectasis
- Tumor growth preserving the parenchymal structures

Reticular Pattern

The reticular pattern is characterized by small and numerous intralobular linear opacities (Table 9.14). As the disease progresses, interlobular septal thickening and traction bronchiectasis are observed.

Honeycombing

It represents a fibrotic and severely damaged lung, characteristic of end-stage lung disease. It presents with multiple well-defined small cysts, from 3–10 mm in size up to 2.5 cm, uniform in size and clustered together. They are associated to traction bronchiectasis (Fig. 9.13).

The diagnosis is challenging as it usually represents an advanced stage of a lung disease and the biopsy is often non-conclusive (Table 9.15).

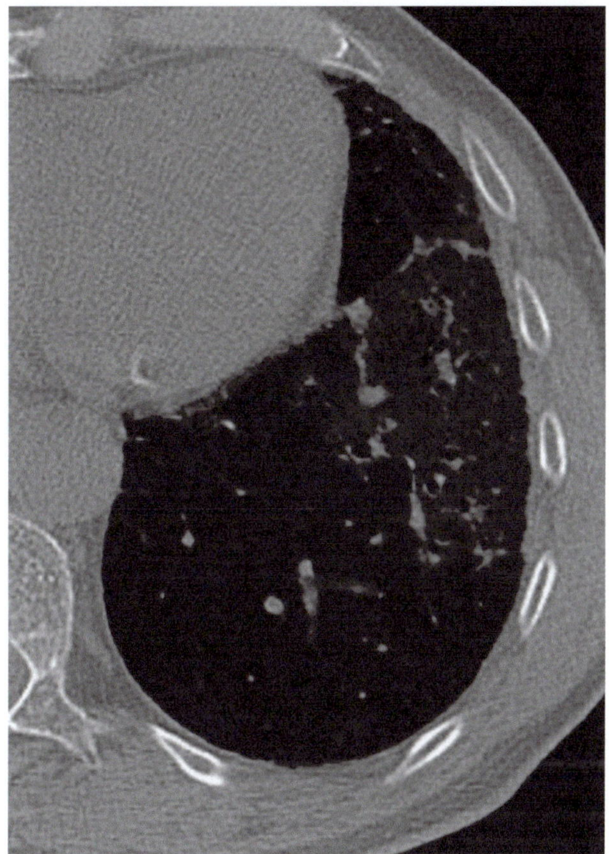

Fig. 9.11 Alveolar pattern. Ground-glass opacity in a patient with NSIP

Table 9.13 Differential diagnosis of alveolar pattern (ground-glass opacity)

Common	
Acute forms	
Atypical pneumonia	Occurs mostly in immunocompromised patients. The most common etiologic agents are P. jirovecii and viral infections (CMV)
Cardiogenic pulmonary edema	Ground-glass opacity with smooth septal thickening, mainly in gravity-dependent regions, associated to pleural effusion
Noncardiogenic pulmonary edema (ARDS)	Ground-glass areas in more than 50% of the lung
Diffuse alveolar hemorrhage	Lobular ground-glass associated to areas of consolidation
Hemorrhagic metastases	Usually secondary to renal cancer
Angioinvasive aspergillosis	Can be associated to ground-glass areas
Hypersensitivity pneumonitis	A mosaic pattern is present in 85% of cases but ground-glass can also be observed

(continued)

Table 9.13 (continued)

Acute eosinophilic pneumonia	Migrating ground-glass opacities with septal thickening and pleural effusion
Drug reaction	Can present in different ways: ARDS, hypersensitivity pneumonitis, pulmonary hemorrhage
Chronic forms	
Non-Specific Interstitial Pneumonia (NSIP)	Can be idiopathic or secondary to scleroderma, rheumatoid arthritis, or drug-induced lung disease It is prevalently characterized by ground-glass, a reticular pattern and traction bronchiectasis. Septal thickening can also be present, more evident at the bases and at the periphery of the lungs. There is subpleural sparing of the lung in the dorsal regions
Chronic eosinophilic pneumonia	Presents with consolidations (100%) and ground-glass appearance (90%) in the peripheral regions and in the upper lobes, with subpleural sparing of the lung
Desquamative Interstitial Pneumonia (DIP)	Of unknown etiology, is more prevalent in heavy smokers. It is characterized by thin-walled cysts (80%), usually in the lower lobes and small in dimension, and ground-glass opacities
Lymphocytic Interstitial Pneumonia (LIP)	Can be idiopathic or secondary to infections (HIV or EBV), dysproteinemia or Sjögren's syndrome. On CT, it appears as thin-walled cysts in 80% of cases, usually less than 20 in number, ground-glass appearance (100%), and nodules in a lymphatic pattern
Primary alveolar proteinosis	The typical presentation is crazy paving pattern, but ground-glass alone may also occur
Less common	
Bronchioloalveolar carcinoma	Focal ground-glass areas not well-defined from surrounding structures or ground-glass associated to solid tissue (part-solid nodule). Air bronchograms may be present
Atypical Adenomatous Hyperplasia (AAH)	Often a precancerous condition. It has a prevalence of 3–7% in the population (higher in elderly patients). It presents as spherical ground-glass opacities that are better delineated than those found in bronchioloalveolar carcinoma

CMV cytomegalovirus, *ARDS* acute respiratory distress syndrome, *HIV* human immunodeficiency virus, *EBV* Epstein–Barr virus

Table 9.14 Differential diagnosis of reticular pattern

Common	
Inferior lung fields	
Idiopathic Pulmonary Fibrosis (IPF)	Idiopathic pathology with a characteristic histopathologic pattern of Usual Interstitial Pneumonia (UIP). The pattern has temporal and spatial heterogeneity. It can be primary (IPF) or secondary to drugs such as chemotherapy, nitrofurantoin, and paraquat The typical radiological presentation is a reticular pattern more evident at the bases and in subpleural regions and traction bronchiectasis with pleural and bronchovascular distortion. It progresses to subpleural honeycombing (multiple rows of cysts, 2–25 mm in size)

Table 9.14 (continued)

Non-Specific Interstitial Pneumonia (NSIP)	Idiopathic or secondary to scleroderma, rheumatoid arthritis, polymyositis, or dermatomyositis. The pattern has temporal and spatial homogeneity The typical radiological presentation is ground-glass opacities that progress to a reticular pattern with septal thickening, which is more evident at the bases and periphery of the lungs. There is sparing of the subpleural lung in dorsal regions. Traction bronchiectasis can also be present, out of proportion to the reticular pattern (Fig. 9.12)
Superior lung fields	
Chronic hypersensitivity pneumonitis	Can mimic IPF and NSIP. It is characterized by a reticular pattern with small fibrous septa that extend from the centrilobular bronchiole to the periphery of the lobule. It has a prevalent involvement of middle portions of the lung in case of chronic exposure (bird fancier's lung); in case of intermittent exposure (farmer's lung), the involvement is more prevalent in the superior portions. Traction bronchiectasis can co-occur (20%)
Sarcoidosis	A reticular pattern may become evident in late stage disease (stage IV) at the level of perihilar regions and in the superior and middle portions of the lung, with distortions and bronchiectasis. The typical presentation is characterized by nodules in a perilymphatic pattern and perihilar and mediastinal adenopathy, which decreases as the fibrosis progresses
Less common	
Asbestosis	Prevalent involvement of the inferior lobes. Pleural plaques may be associated
Ankylosing spondylitis	Prevalent involvement of the superior lobes
Lymphangitic carcinomatosis	Usually presents with a septal pattern but can mimic a reticular one. It is characterized by an asymmetric involvement of one or more lobes

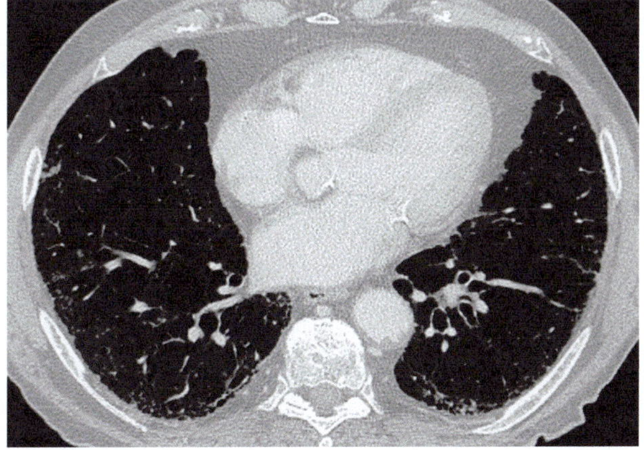

Fig. 9.12 Reticular pattern in a patient with NSIP

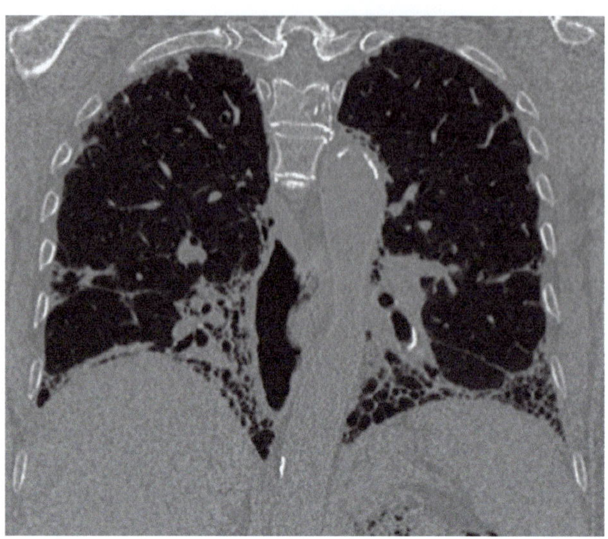

Fig. 9.13 Honeycombing in a patient with IPF

Table 9.15 Differential diagnosis of honeycombing

Common	
Inferior lung fields	
Idiopathic Pulmonary Fibrosis (IPF)	Always evolves into honeycombing
Non-Specific Interstitial Pneumonia (NSIP)	On CT it progresses to honeycombing only rarely but on histologic examination the so-called microscopic honeycombing is observed frequently
Asbestosis	Presents, similarly to IPF, the histological pattern of UIP. Its distinguishing features are pleural plaques (80%), fibrosis centered at the respiratory bronchiole (where the fibers deposit) and ramifying towards the pleura, peripheral hump- or wedge-shaped homogeneous opacities due to the obstruction of the respiratory bronchioles, lobular air-trapping (infrequent in IPF). Infrequently, it progresses to honeycombing
Superior lung fields	
Stage IV sarcoidosis	Can cause honeycombing prevalently in the superior lobes. Fibrous bands are present from the hilum along the bronchovascular bundles
Chronic hypersensitivity pneumonitis	Honeycombing can develop in the superior and middle regions, with relative basal sparing. Centrilobular nodules (not common in IPF) and lobular air-trapping (not common in IPF) can co-occur
Less common diagnoses	
Ionizing radiations	Secondary to thoracic radiotherapy
Diffuse alveolar damage (ARDS)	Occurs secondary to the fibrotic repair response to an acute damage and after the barotrauma occurring in the setting of positive-pressure ventilation

Suggested Readings

Hansell DM, et al. CT staging and monitoring of fibrotic interstitial lung diseases in clinical practice and treatment trials: a position paper from the Fleischner Society. Lancet Respir Med. 2015;3(6):483–96.

Dalpiaz G. Cancellieri A. Atlas of Diffuse Ling Diseases: A Multidisciplinary Approach. Editor: Springer 2017.

Mueller-Mang C, et al. What every radiologist should know about idiopathic interstitial pneumonia. Radiographics. 2007;27:595–615.

Nishino HM, et al. A practical approach to high-resolution CT of diffuse lung disease. Eur J Radiol. 2014;83(1):6–19.

Pleural Diseases

10

Vincenzo Noce and Rosa Maria Ammendola

When approaching pleural diseases the first step is to correctly determine whether the pathological finding has a pleural or extrapleural origin. This discrimination could be challenging since pleural diseases may have an intraparenchymal extension and vice versa. A simple diagnostic sign to correctly identify the anatomical characteristics of the expanding mass consists into studying the angle formed with the surface of origin. When at the lesion base the angle is obtuse, it originates from the pleural plane; instead, if the angle is acute, it arises from the lung parenchyma and infiltrates or contacts the pleura only later (Fig. 10.1).

Independently from the etiology, pleural diseases can manifest with four principal patterns: effusion, pneumothorax, thickening, and masses.

Pleural Effusion

Fluid accumulation in the pleural cavity can be determined by several causes. From a clinical and cytological point of view we can distinguish transudate and exudate fluid. Transudate has low protein content (less than 3 g/dL), is frequently the result of systemic pathological processes and is more often bilateral. Exudate has high protein content (more than 3 g/dL) and is secondary to local irritating factors.

On CXR the possibility to observe an effusion depends on the amount of fluid present and the patient's position. When the patient is in the upright position, a small effusion collects in the posterobasal regions. On LL view it appears as a blunting of the posterior costophrenic angle; on PA view, it may be more complex to identify the fluid, but it is possible to appreciate its presence indirectly as an elevation and lateralization of the hemidiaphragmatic dome on the affected side ("pseudo-diaphragm" sign; Fig. 10.2a). Larger quantities of fluid present with a Damoiseau-Ellis line

V. Noce · R. M. Ammendola (✉)
Department of Radiological, Oncological and Pathological Sciences, Sapienza University of Rome, Rome, Italy

I. Carbone, M. Anzidei (eds.), *Thoracic Radiology*,
https://doi.org/10.1007/978-3-030-35765-8_10

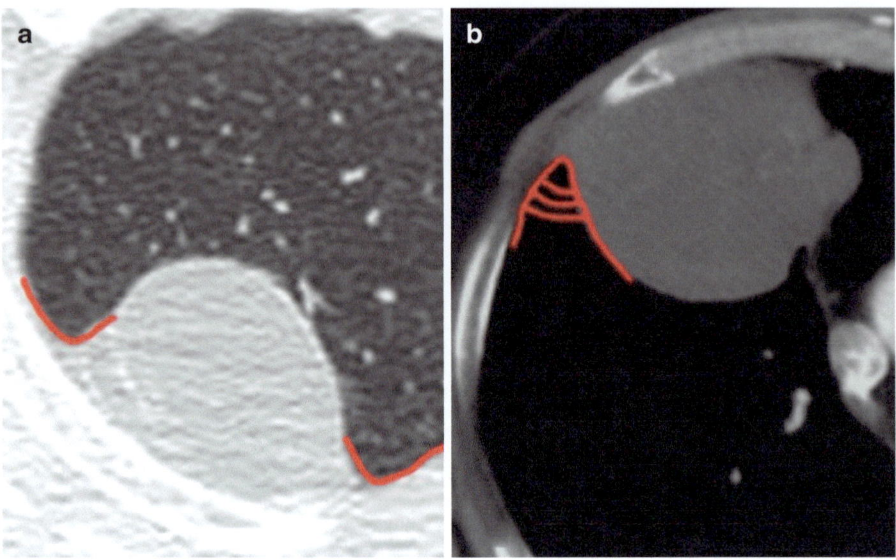

Fig. 10.1 (**a**) Pleural lesion forming obtuse angles with the pleura, (**b**) Pulmonary lesion, forming an acute angle with the pleura

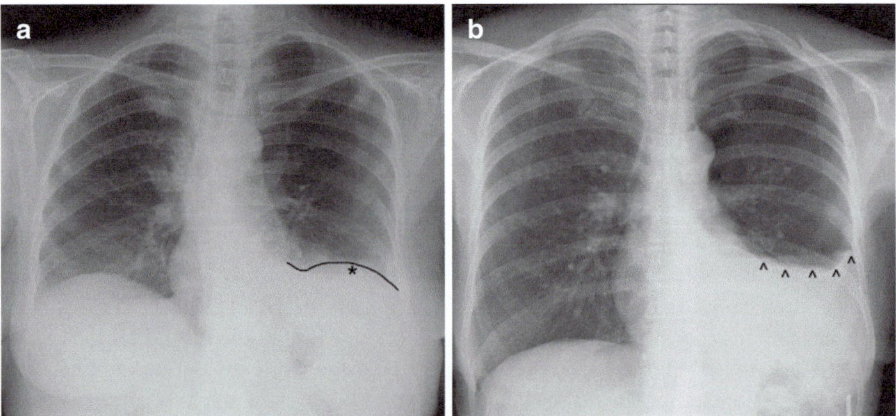

Fig. 10.2 (**a**) Pseudo-diaphragm sign (*), characteristic of a mild/moderate amount of fluid, (**b**) Damoiseau-Ellis line (^), observed in larger effusions

(Fig. 10.2b), a contralateral shift of the mediastinal structures and the accumulation of fluid within fissures in the LL view. In a supine patient the fluid collects mostly in the posterior regions in a gravity-dependent pattern. Therefore, it may be difficult to observe on chest X-ray, where it appears as a loss of the hemidiaphragm silhouette or blunting of the lateral costophrenic angles (with larger effusions).

A CT scan is more accurate for identifying pleural effusion, allowing a more precise estimate of its quantity and an immediate visualization of possible associated findings (pleural thickenings, cardiovascular anomalies, etc.).

The empyema is caused by the accumulation of purulent material within the pleural space. It manifests as a loculated effusion with lenticular shape, forming an obtuse angle with the pleural surface. Contrast-enhanced CT scan allows to visualize the vascularization of the expanding pathologic process and inflammatory processes in the adjacent soft tissues.

Pneumothorax

Pneumothorax refers to the presence of air in the pleural space. The air localizes anteriorly and over the diaphragm, with its distribution depending on the position of the patient and the presence of pleural adhesions. When there is a clinical suspicion of pneumothorax (history of thoracic trauma and/or suggestive clinical findings), the first-line exam is a CXR, which is accurate and easy to perform also in urgency or emergency conditions. In a standing CXR, the pneumothorax appears as a crescent-shaped radiolucency with no lung markings that causes a contralateral shift of the mediastinal structures. Occasionally, a radio-opaque line may underline the radiolucent pleural space (visceral pleura sign; Fig. 10.3a).

In the supine patient, the pneumothorax may be more difficult to identify, presenting as an air collection in the costophrenic angles, delimited by the diaphragm and the mediastinal structures (deep sulcus sign; Fig. 10.3b).

A CT scan is usually required in case of diagnostic doubts on the CXR or in case of recurrent pneumothorax of unknown etiology.

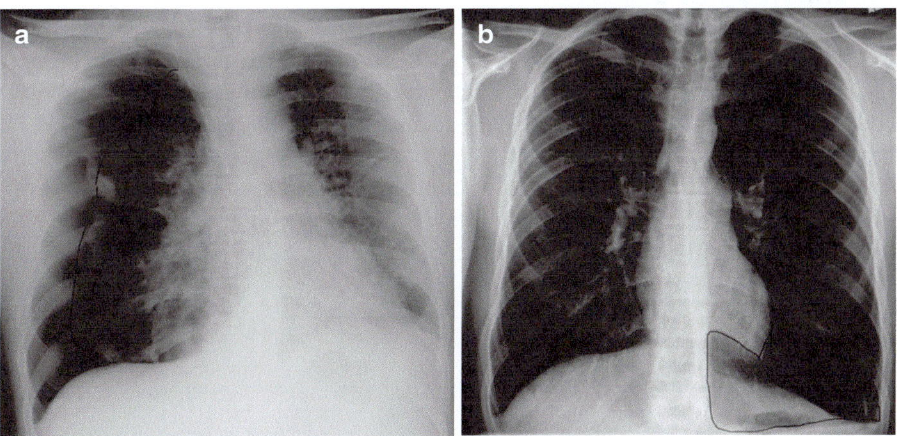

Fig. 10.3 Distribution of the air (outlined) within the pleural cavity in a standing patient (**a**) and air localized within the costophrenic angle (**b**)

Pleural Thickenings and Masses

Pleural thickenings and masses are pathologic findings characterized by the presence of solid tissue (inflammatory, fibrous, or neoplastic) within the pleural space. Based on the extent of pleural involvement, it is possible to distinguish a mass (focal) from a thickening (diffuse).

For pleural thickening inferior to 1 cm associated to a pleural effusion, the CT is able to provide information only on the exudative nature of the effusion but is not enough to associate this finding to a specific pleural pathology.

Pleural fibrosis frequently results from scar formation after a previous pleural infectious disease, especially if purulent. Pleural fibrosis often manifests as a focal thickening, with regular and well-defined margins, and is better identified on a CT scan. When it occurs in the posterior costophrenic angles, it cannot be distinguished from a small pleural effusion.

Pleural plaques are acellular collagenous matrix deposits, sometimes with calcium salts inclusions. They are typically associated to asbestos exposure, and their extension correlates with the intensity of the chronic inhalation. Typical imaging finding are the greater vertical extension, parallel to the ribs. They may affect the diaphragmatic pleura, sparing the apices and the costophrenic angles. Furthermore, pleural asbestosis is associated to the development of round atelectasis.

A diffuse fibrotic thickening can be secondary to asbestosis or hemothorax, massive infectious pleurisy (often tubercular), and empyema. On imaging, there is a pronounced pleural thickening, often associated to coarse calcifications and a significant loss of volume of the affected hemithorax. These findings can be indicative of significant morbidity as they may result into pronounced ventilation deficits.

Pleural Neoplasia

Pleural neoplasia can be primary (solitary fibrous tumor of the pleura, malignant pleural mesothelioma) or secondary (metastases from pulmonary, breast or thoracic soft tissue tumors), both commonly associated to pleural effusion. In 80–90% of cases the cytology exam of pleural fluid is positive for neoplastic cells. Pleural metastases from breast and lung cancer are the most common etiologies of malignant pleural effusions. A circumferential pleural thickening, nodular or more than 1 cm thick, is highly suggestive of pleural neoplasia.

Mesothelioma

The mesothelioma is a primary pleural neoplasia with poor prognosis, strongly correlated to asbestos exposure (5% prevalence in the exposed population). The epithelioid histotype (50% of the cases) has a better prognosis and is accompanied by abundant pleural effusions. Instead, the sarcomatoid histotype (25% of the cases) is characterized by poor or absent effusions.

Usually, the mesothelioma spreads by direct continuity to the pleura and adjacent fissures; hematogenous spread may occur in 50% of cases. On chest X-ray the most common finding is a pleural effusion, possibly with the presence of a circumferential or lobulated pleural thickening, which represents a solid pleural mass or a loculated effusion (Fig. 10.4).

A typical sign is the so-called frozen mediastinum sign, defined as the lack of mediastinal shift even with massive unilateral effusion. This is provoked by a diffuse pleural infiltration, involving also the mediastinal side. On chest CT pleural effusion and pleural thickening are present in the 75% and in 90% of cases, respectively. The typical thickening in mesothelioma is circumferential, continuous, and nodular. In the early phases of the disease, the thickening may be regular and discontinuous (Fig. 10.5).

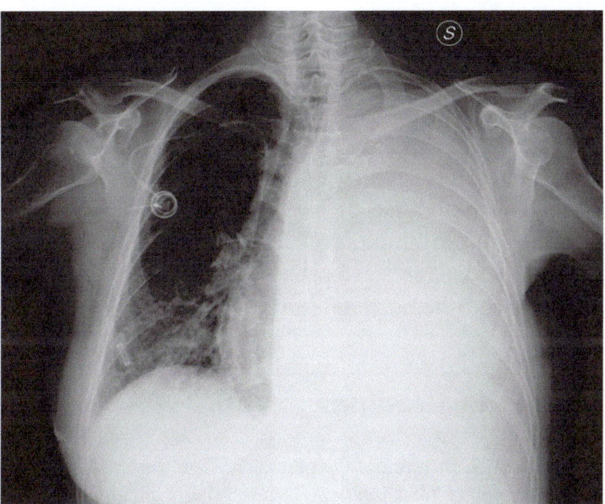

Fig. 10.4 Left massive pleural effusion in a patient with mesothelioma

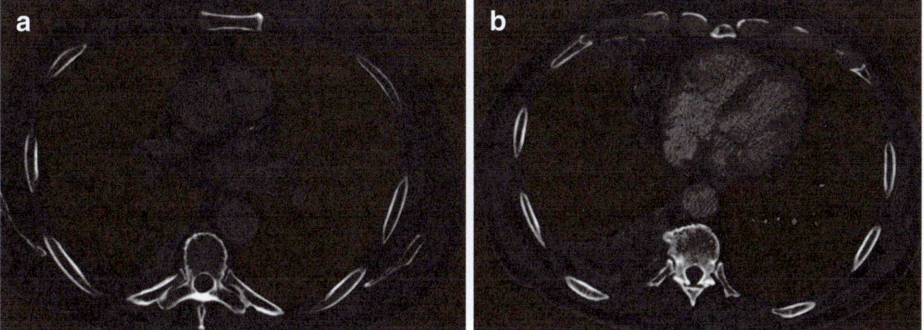

Fig. 10.5 CT scan in a patient with mesothelioma: pleural effusion (**a**, **b**) associated to a vascularized solid thickening of the outer and inner pleura (**b**)

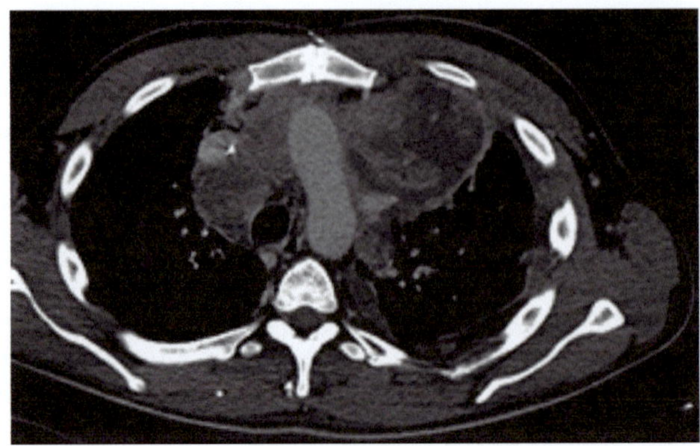

Fig. 10.6 Solid, nodular, pleural lesions secondary to thymic neoplasia

Pleural Metastases

The most common neoplasia metastasizing to the pleura are adenocarcinomas (more than 40% lung cancer, 20% breast cancer, ovarian cancer, lymphoma, stomach cancer).

A pleural effusion is almost always appreciable. The pleural thickening can be linear, macronodular, or circumferential. Pleural carcinomatosis defines a diffuse, multinodular infiltration of the pleura (Fig. 10.6). This condition is the manifestation of a very aggressive process and is often secondary to breast cancer and associated to a sero-hemorrhagic exudate.

Suggested Readings

Helm EJ, et al. Imaging of the pleura. J Magn Reson Imaging. 2010;32(6):1275–86.

Kuhlman JE, et al. Complex disease of the pleural space: radiographic and CT evaluation. Radiographics. 1997;17:63–79.

Qureshi NR, et al. Imaging of pleural disease. Clin Chest Med. 2006;27(2):193–213.

Vascular Diseases of the Thorax

11

Federica Ciolina

Introduction

Computed Tomography Angiography (CTA) is used both in emergency settings to identify acute pathologies such as acute aortic syndromes and in routine clinical practice to detect or monitor aortic diseases and to identify acute pulmonary embolism. It is a fast and easily available procedure, thanks to its high temporal and spatial resolution and to the widespread availability on the territory, providing a panoramic view of the entire cardiopulmonary structures. Moreover, the volumetric acquisition allows to obtain multiplanar reconstruction (MPR) and three-dimensional volume rendering (3D-VR) that make CTA the main reference for treatment planning.

Magnetic Resonance Imaging (MRI), being less invasive, can be considered a valid alternative to monitor known and stationary aortic diseases, and it is the preferred methodology for pediatric patients.

Anatomy and Anatomical Variants of the Aorta

The aorta consists of three different portions: the aortic root, the aortic arch, and the descending portion.

1. The aortic root consists of:
   (a) the aortic annulus, which is a fibrous ring that anchors the aortic valve. It is at the origin of the outflow tract from the left ventricle.

F. Ciolina (✉)
Department of Radiological, Oncological and Pathological Sciences, Sapienza University of Rome, Rome, Italy

I. Carbone, M. Anzidei (eds.), *Thoracic Radiology*,
https://doi.org/10.1007/978-3-030-35765-8_11

(b) the aortic bulb, which is the junction between the left ventricular outflow tract and the aorta.
(c) the sinotubular junction, which is the transition between the bulbar and tubular portion of the ascending aorta.

Distal to the aortic root there are:

2. the ascending aorta
3. the aortic arch with the origin of epiaortic vessels
4. the isthmus, which is the physiological narrowing of the aortic diameter distal to the origin of the left subclavian artery
5. the descending thoracic aorta

Aortic anatomy is summarized in Fig. 11.1.

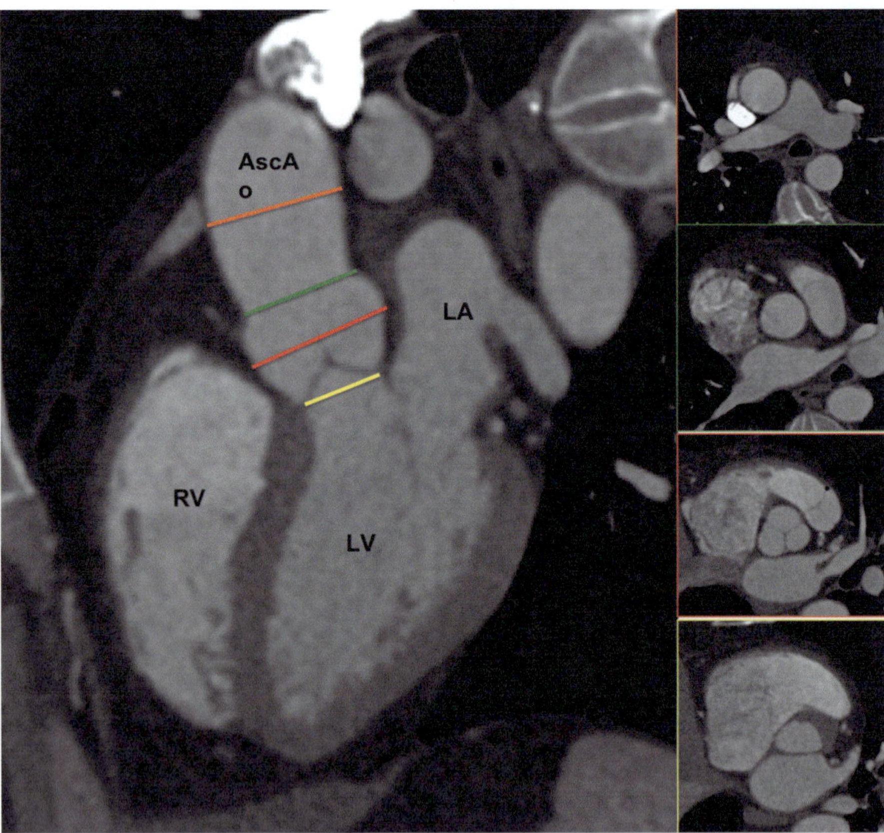

Fig. 11.1 Normal anatomy of the aortic root. *AscAo* ascending aorta, *LA* left atrium, *LV* left ventricle, *RV* right ventricle

The anatomical variants of the thoracic aorta usually occur at the aortic arch and can be modifications in the morphology and course of the aorta and anomalies at the origin of the branches of the aortic arch. These variants are usually seen incidentally in healthy people (25%) and are not clinically significant. In 80% of cases, the anomaly is the origin of the left common carotid artery from the anonymous trunk (bovine arch) (Fig. 11.2). Less common anomalies are: a separate origin of the four aortic branches from the arch, the origin of an isolated vertebral artery from the arch, or the retroesophageal course of the subclavian artery (lusory artery) (Fig. 11.3).

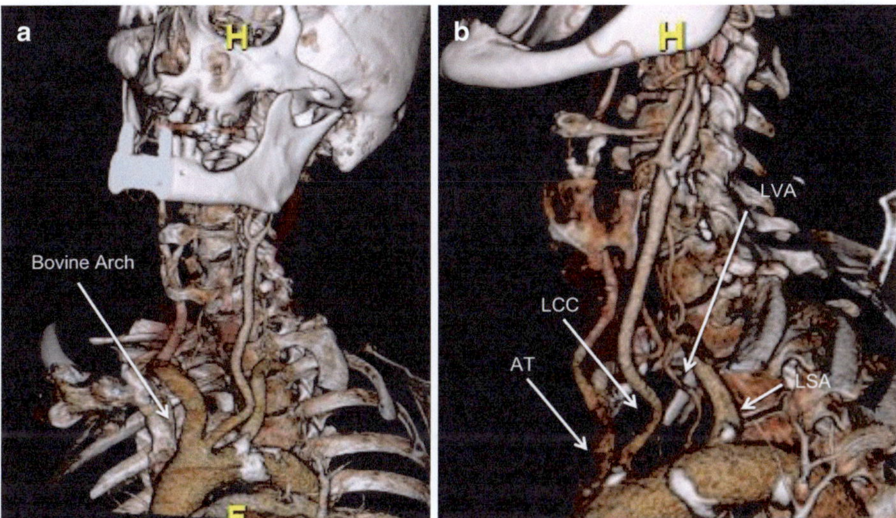

Fig. 11.2 (**a**) Bovine arch: the anonymous artery and the right common carotid artery originate from a single trunk, (**b**) Origin of the left vertebral artery directly from the aortic arch. *AT* anonymous trunk, *LCC* left common carotid artery, *LVA* left vertebral artery, *LSA* left subclavian artery

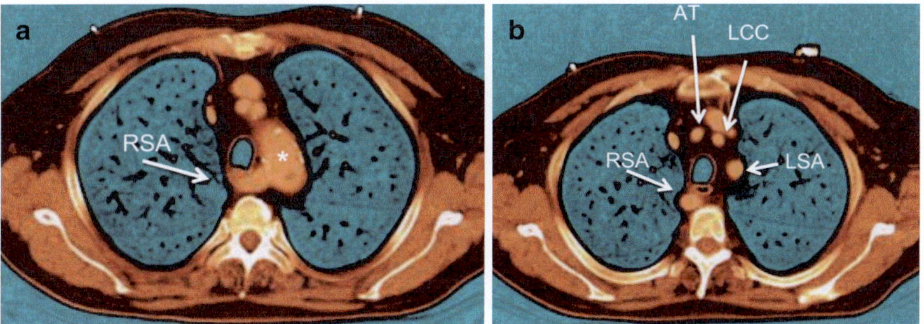

Fig. 11.3 Lusory artery. (**a**) The right subclavian artery (*RSA*) originates as the last vessel from the aortic arch (*white asterisk*) and goes from left to right passing behind the trachea and the esophagus (**b**). *AT* anonymous trunk, *LCC* left common carotid artery, *LSA* left subclavian artery

Anatomy and Anatomical Variants of the Pulmonary Arteries and Veins

The anatomy of the pulmonary arteries and veins is shown in Figs. 11.4 and 11.5.

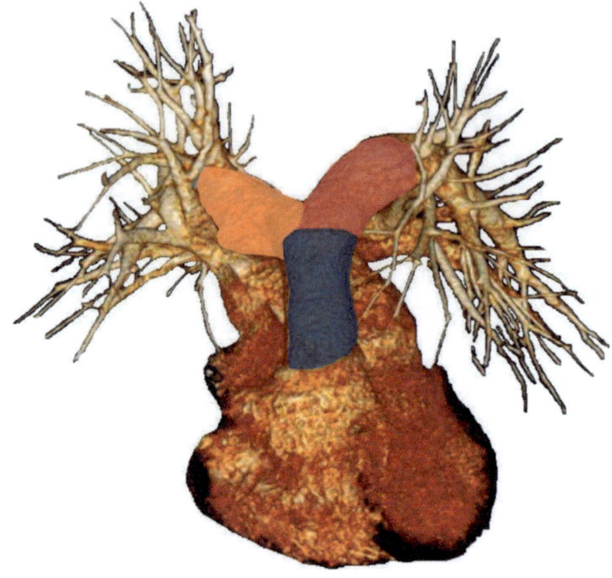

Fig. 11.4 Normal anatomy of the pulmonary arteries: in *blue* the main trunk, in *orange* the right pulmonary artery, in *red* the left pulmonary artery. (*From Napoli A, Ciolina F, Bertaccini L. Pulmonary Circulation. In: Catalano C, Anzidei M, Napoli A (eds) Cardiovascular CT and MR imaging. Milan: Springer; 2013, with permission*)

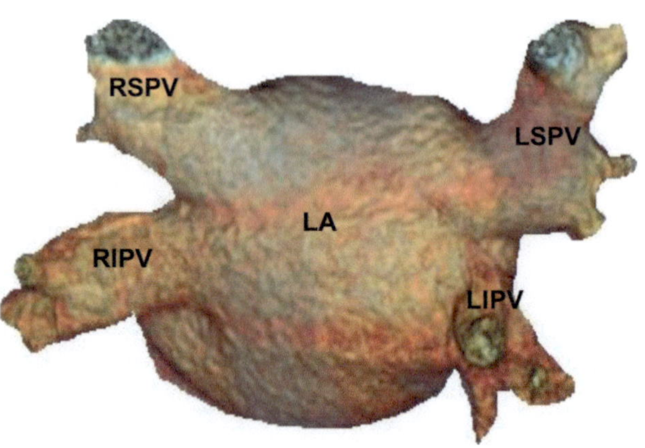

Fig. 11.5 Normal anatomy of the pulmonary veins. Posterior view of the left atrium (*LA*): usually two veins drain the right lung and two the left lung. *RSPV* right superior pulmonary vein, *RIPV* right inferior pulmonary vein, *LSPV* left superior pulmonary vein, *LIPV* left inferior pulmonary vein. (*From Napoli A, Ciolina F, Bertaccini L. Pulmonary circulation. In: Catalano C, Anzidei M, Napoli A (eds) Cardiovascular CT and MR imaging. Milan: Springer; 2013, with permission*)

The main anatomic variants of the arterial pulmonary system are:

- *Congenital hypoplasia of the pulmonary artery*: it is the most common congenital anatomical variant and consists in a reduced caliber of the lobar and segmental branches of the pulmonary artery without the involvement of the main trunk. Symptoms are related to overload of the right heart; follow-up is suggested for evaluation during growth. Patients with advanced symptoms require lung transplant.
- *Anomalous origin of the left pulmonary artery*: it is a rare vascular developmental anomaly in which there is a regression of the left pulmonary artery during embryonic life. Thus, the left artery arises from the posterior portion of the right pulmonary artery and passes between the trachea and esophagus to reach the left hilum. It may be isolated and often asymptomatic or may be associated with other cardiovascular and bronchial anomalies (15%). It has a high mortality and morbidity rate during childhood. Treatment is surgical, consisting in the ligation of the vessel with re-implantation in the correct position.

Pulmonary veins are usually four (a superior and an inferior vein from each lung). There can be numerical anomalies or anomalous venous returns, such as Partial Anomalous Pulmonary Venous Return (PAPVR) or Total Anomalous Pulmonary Venous Return (TAPVR).

- *PAPVR* is a pulmonary-to-systemic left-to-right shunt caused by drainage of one or more pulmonary veins into the right heart or into a great venous vessel (i.e., superior vena cava, azygos vein, venous brachiocephalic trunk, inferior vena cava, or coronary sinus) that drains into the right atrium.
- *TAPVR* is a rare anomaly (2% of cardiac malformations) occurring when the pulmonary veins fail to drain into the left atrium and form an unusual connection with some other cardiovascular structure. It can be classified into four types. Survival is possible only in the presence of an atrial septal defect or a patent foramen ovale that causes a right-to-left shunt.

Congenital Aortic Malformations

During the embryological and fetal life, the arterial vascular anatomy consists of a ventral trunk which splits into two arches and rejoins into a single dorsal trunk. Congenital aortic malformations are derived from an abnormal regression of the right arch between the origin of the ipsilateral subclavian artery and the junction with the left arch and can result into the persistence of a complete vascular ring (double aortic arch) or a right-sided aortic arch. This last is generated from the obliteration of the left arch, with the presence of a left anonymous trunk (mirror image branching) or left retroesophageal subclavian artery (lusory). These anomalies may be asymptomatic or clinically relevant due to the compression of the trachea and/or esophagus (dysphagia, dyspnea, respiratory infections), and they are in many cases associated with other congenital cardiovascular abnormalities.

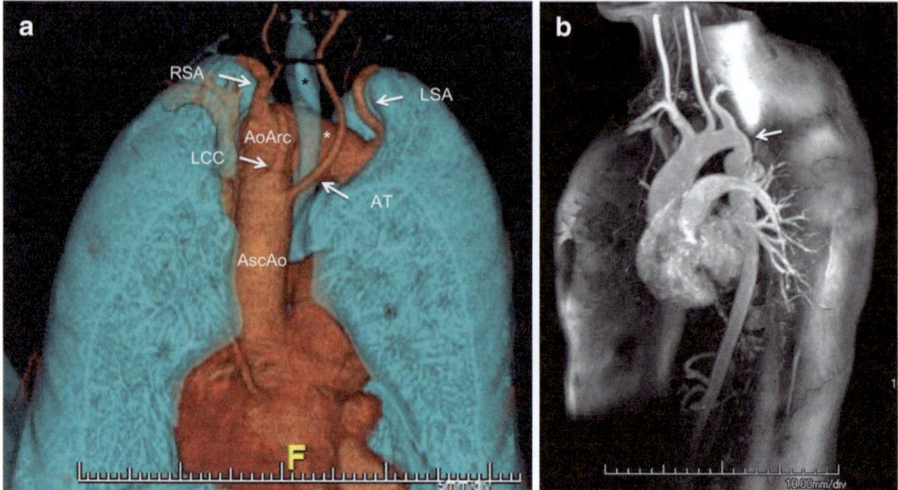

Fig. 11.6 (**a**) Kommerell diverticulum (*white asterisk*): dilatation of right-sided aortic arc with left subclavian artery originating from the diverticulum as the last vessel, (**b**) Coarctation of the aorta with narrowing at the level of the aortic isthmus (*white arrow*). *AscAo* ascending aorta, *AoArc* aortic arch; trachea (*black asterisk*), *AT* anonymous trunk, *LCC* left common carotid artery, *RSA* right subclavian artery, *LSA*, left subclavian artery

Kommerell diverticulum consists in an aneurysmal dilation of the origin of the aberrant subclavian artery, determined by atresia of the portion of the contralateral arch between the origin of the carotid artery and the subclavian artery often associated with a right-sided arch (Fig. 11.6a).

Botallo duct is a small arterial duct connecting the pulmonary artery and the aorta: it allows blood circulation during fetal life and normally obliterates spontaneously after birth, as it is no longer necessary. It can persist, becoming clinically relevant only when it leads to a hemodynamically significant shunt.

Coarctation of the aorta is a congenital narrowing of the aorta at the level of the aortic isthmus, often associated with bicuspid aortic valve, ventricular septal defect, or other congenital anomalies (Fig. 11.6b). Symptoms depend on the development of collateral circulation through the internal mammary artery, intercostal arteries, thyrocervical or costocervical trunks.

Acute Aortic Syndromes

Acute aortic syndromes are a group of life-threatening pathological conditions (aortic dissection, intramural hematoma, or penetrating aortic ulcer) of degenerative or traumatic origin with overlapping symptoms, usually characterized by intense chest pain, that is sometimes irradiated to the back, or syncope (Fig. 11.7).

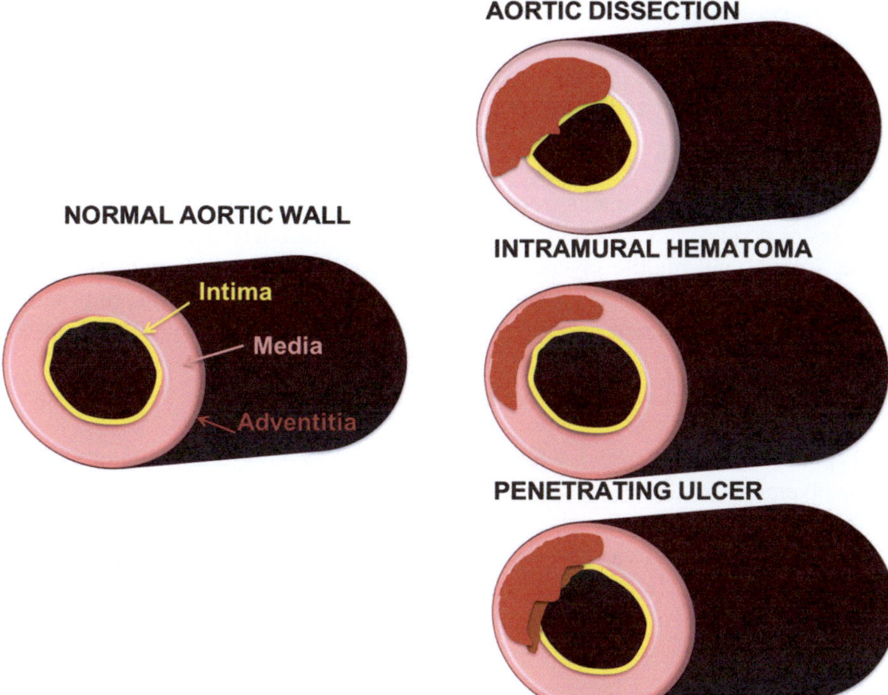

Fig. 11.7 Pathogenesis of acute aortic syndromes. In aortic dissection, there is an intimal tear with extravasation of blood within the media. Intramural hematoma is a spontaneous hemorrhage of the vasa vasorum of the tunica media which weakens the media without an intimal tear. Penetrating ulcer occurs in the presence of ulceration of an atheromatous plaque that disrupts the inner, elastic layer of the aortic wall, reaches the tunica media, and forms a hematoma in the media

Predisposing factors are hypertension (70%), old age, atherosclerosis, previous surgery, cardiac surgery, congenital disorders (Marfan syndrome, Ehlers-Danlos syndrome, Turner syndrome), and congenital heart defects (coarctation).

When acute aortic disease is suspected, an early diagnosis is needed to select the appropriate treatment. CT scan is the recommended initial examination. MRI has a minor role, being indicated only in subacute cases with stable clinical conditions or during follow-up when close monitoring is required, in order to reduce dose-cumulative radiation and kidney damage by iodinated contrast media. In the image acquisition protocol, a pre-contrast scan must always be included. ECG-gating is needed to avoid pulsing artifacts if involvement of the ascending aorta is suspected, and when the coronary arteries are to be evaluated (triple rule-out).

Aortic Dissection

Acute aortic dissection is the most common cause of aortic emergency. Its prevalence exceeds that of thoracoabdominal aortic aneurysm rupture. It is due to a tear in the tunica intima, which results in the formation of two lumina (a false lumen and a true lumen).

Aortic dissection originates from a combination of congenital connective tissue diseases or acquired factors (atherosclerosis), which can determine the weakening of the intimal and middle layers of the aortic wall. Traumatic or microtraumatic events can damage the intima. Otherwise, a hematoma of the vasa vasorum within the aortic wall can stretch and crack the intima by increasing the pressure in the middle layer.

It can be classified according to Stanford classification in:

- Type A (60–70% of cases), when it involves the ascending aorta with or without involvement of the descending aorta, regardless of the location of the tear (Fig. 11.8).
- Type B (30–40% of cases), when the tear is located distal to the origin of the anonymous trunk. It may involve the aortic arch and/or the descending aorta, but always spares the ascending aorta (Fig. 11.9).

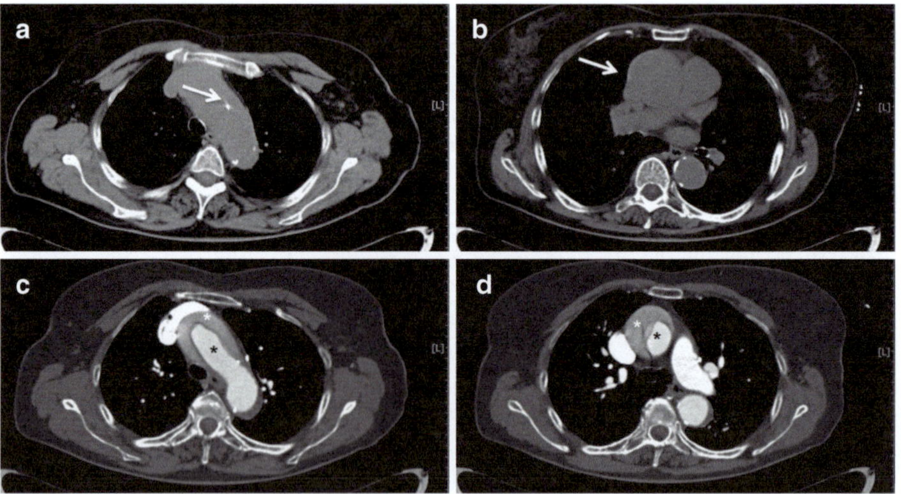

Fig. 11.8 Type A aortic dissection. (**a**) Intimal calcification (arrow), (**b**) Hyperattenuation in the ascending aorta, (**c**, **d**) True lumen (*black asterisk*), and false lumen (*white asterisk*) separated by the intima

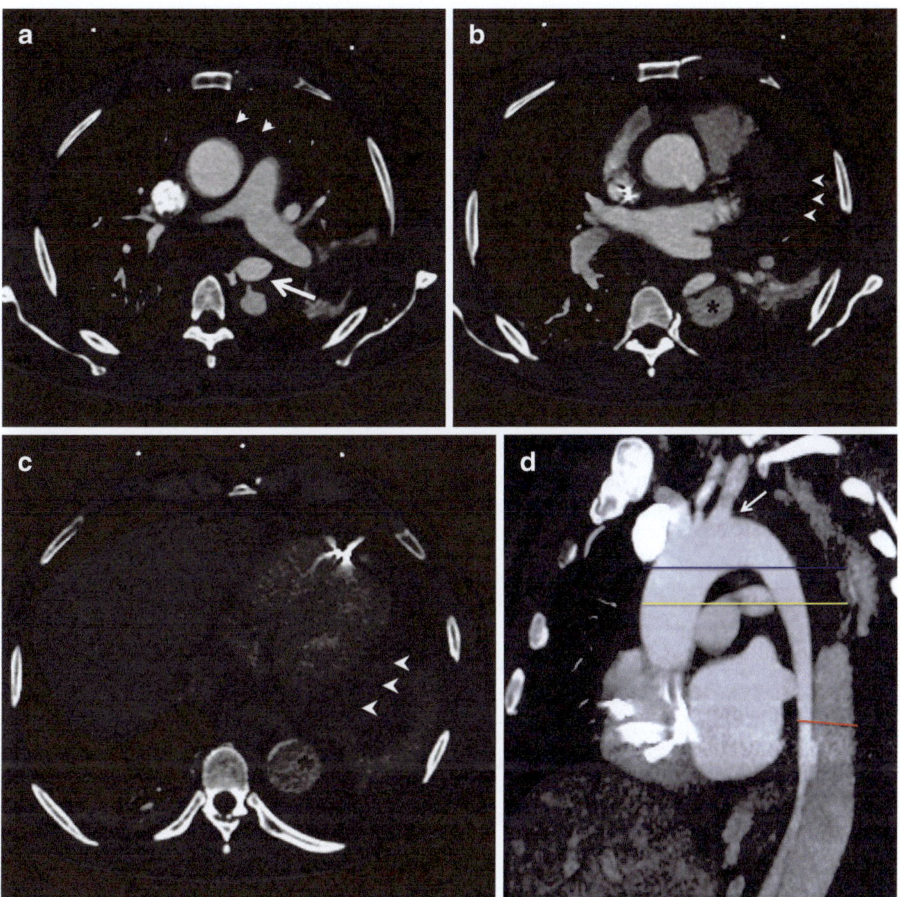

Fig. 11.9 Type B aortic dissection. (**a**) Tear in the descending aorta (*Blu level*), (**b**, **c**) Different dimension of false lumen (*black asterisk*) and true lumen due to pulsation. There is pericardial effusion (*white arrowheads*) and pleural effusion (*black arrow head*). (**d**) Sagittal MPR of thoracic aorta

Thoracic aortic dissection may be described as acute or chronic, depending on the clinical manifestations: it is acute if symptoms have been present for less than 2 weeks, chronic if they have been present for 2 weeks or longer (Fig. 11.10).

Stanford type A requires urgent cardiac surgery, while Stanford type B needs medical (antihypertensive medications) or endovascular treatment (if there is an aortic lumen >6 cm, hemodynamic instability, complications or progression of dissection, pain persistence, or organ ischemia). In case of chronic or stable dissections, follow-up with CTA or MRA at 1, 3, 6, and 12 months and then every 6 months is indicated.

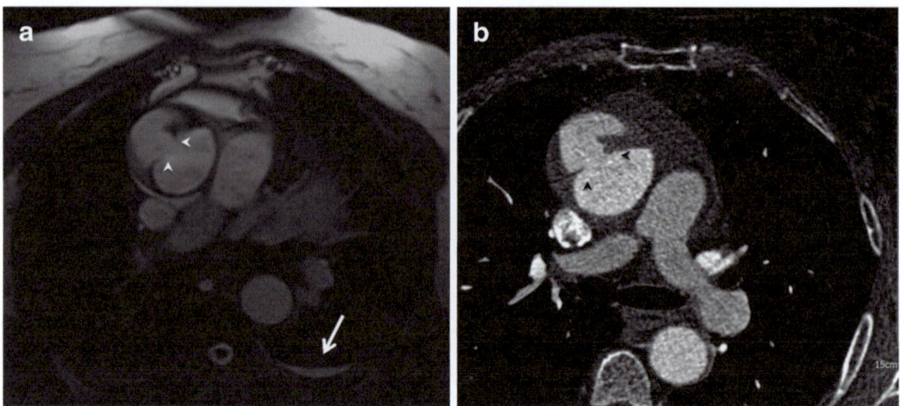

Fig. 11.10 78-year-old woman presenting to the Emergency Department with chest pain. Takotsubo syndrome was suspected and an MR was performed to study the left ventricle. (**a**) On TRUFI axial images of the thorax, an intimal tear (*arrowheads*) and pleural effusion (*white arrow*) are evident, (**b**) CT confirms type A aortic dissection

Complications may be aortic rupture (78% of untreated cases), hemothorax, mediastinal hematoma, hemopericardium with cardiac tamponade, hematoma around the pulmonary branches, and aortic regurgitation with acute heart failure. It can also cause compression of the arterial branches (20% of cases), resulting in myocardial infarction (if the coronary arteries are compressed), stroke, spinal cord ischemia, renal or upper limb or abdominal organ ischemia.

- *Pre-contrast CT findings:*
  - Calcifications
  - Intramural hematoma
  - Hemomediastinum
  - Pleural effusion, pericardial effusion, or hemopericardium (Fig. 11.11)
- *Post-contrast CT findings:*
  - Dissection type (A or B)
  - Localization of intimal tear
  - Rupture
  - Intramural hematoma
  - Thrombosis of the true or false lumen (usually the false lumen is prone to thrombosis, is less bright and bigger than the true lumen, and forms an acute angle with the aortic wall)
  - Compression of the true or false lumen
  - Involvement of aortic valve or coronary arteries in type A
  - Involvement of epiaortic or splanchnic vessels and perfusion of abdominal organs
  - Vessels stenosis, compression, or occlusion

In case a type A dissection is suspected, ECG-gating should be used; to diagnose or control type B dissection, cardiac gating is not necessary (Fig. 11.12).

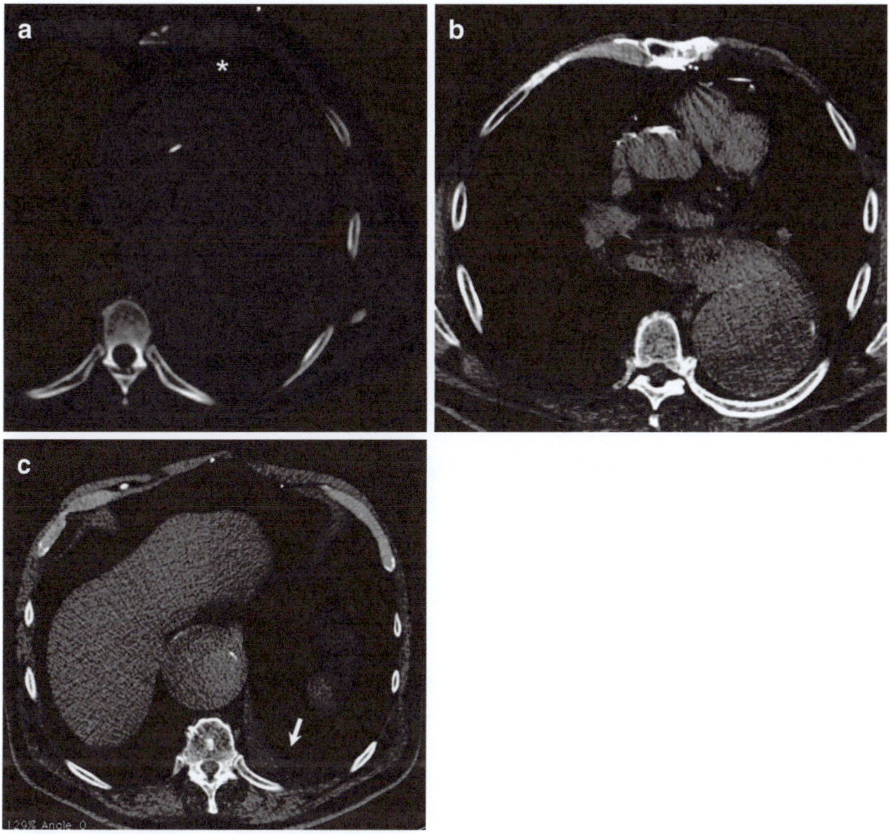

Fig. 11.11 (**a**) Hemopericardium, (**b**) Hemomediastinum, (**c**) Pleural effusion

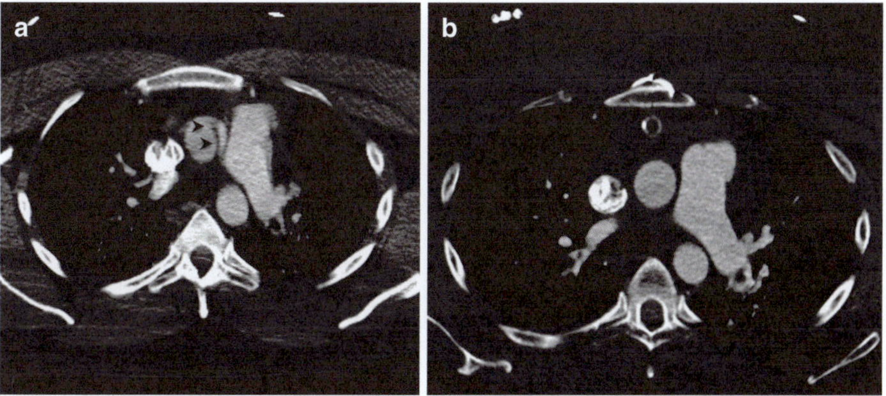

Fig. 11.12 30-year-old man presenting to the Emergency Department after a car accident. (**a**) CT scan was done without ECG-gating and a type A dissection was suspected, (**b**) After cardiothoracic surgery that had not found the dissection, CT was repeated using ECG-gating

- *MRI scan:*

  T1- and T2-weighted pre-contrast sequences are acquired to detect intramural hematoma or the false lumen of dissection; serial contrast-enhanced GRE (GRadient Echo) sequences are necessary to assess the dynamics of contrast agent (if available, time-resolved technique).
- *MRI findings:*
  - *TSE (Turbo Spin Echo) sequences*: In T1-weighted sequences, there is hypointense or intermediate signal intensity in case of communication with the circulating blood (oxyhemoglobin signal) and in case of high-flow supply of the false lumen (flow-void artifact). Hyperintensity of the false lumen indicates methemoglobin presence and can be helpful to distinguish acute from chronic blood. On T2-weighted images, the false lumen is hyperintense compared to the true lumen if there is thrombosis or slow flow (Fig. 11.13).

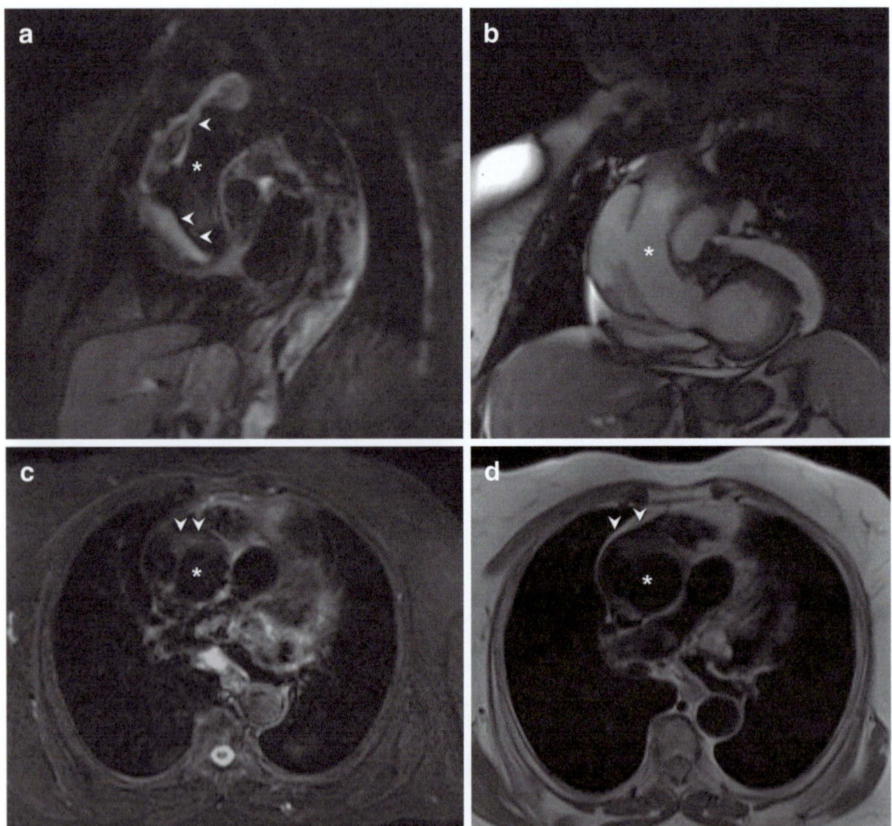

Fig. 11.13 (**a**, **c**)*:* T2-STIR image shows hyperintensity of the false lumen (*arrowheads*). (**d**) T1-weighted image shows hypointensity or intermediate signal intensity of the false lumen (*arrowheads*) due to communication with the circulating blood (oxyhemoglobin signal) and to high-flow supply of the false lumen (flow-void artifact), as showed in coronal view (**b**). *White asterisk*, true lumen

- *SSFP (Steady-State Free Precession) sequences*: In the cine images, the intimal flap shifts consensually to the pulsation, the flow is turbulent in the false lumen and accelerated in the true lumen.
- *PC (Phase Contrast) velocity-encoded sequences:* these allow to detect the direction of the flow in the false lumen.
- *Contrast-enhanced GRE sequences*: they highlight the differences between the two lumens in terms of morphology and size and they study the contrast media dynamics. False lumen will have a delayed filling compared to the true lumen (serial sequence).

Intramural Hematoma (IMH)

It is caused by a spontaneous hemorrhage of the vasa vasorum of the middle layer, which weakens the media without an intimal tear.

It can be classified using Stanford type A (57%) and type B (43%) as for aortic dissection.

The evolution is variable: it may result into aortic rupture (adventitial side breach), evolve into aortic dissection (16–47%, secondary intimal break) or aneurysm formation (for weakening of the aortic wall), or it can stabilize, regress, or spontaneously resolve (especially if involves only the descending aorta).

- On pre-contrast CT scan, IMH appears as a crescent-shaped area of attenuation in the aortic wall (i.e., the hematoma in the middle layer), which may or may not compress the aortic lumen. In IMH, there is also an abnormal circumferential thickening of the aortic wall (variable thickness from 3 mm to 1 cm, it is diagnostic if thickness >7 mm with a density >60 HU). Moreover, IMH may displace intimal calcifications.

  When aortic dissection is suspected, it is mandatory to perform unenhanced CT as the first imaging evaluation because contrast material within the vessel may obscure IMH (Fig. 11.14).
- On post-contrast CT scan, no intimal tears are visible and the crescent-shaped area is not perfused by contrast. The course is circumferential (in dissection, it shows a spiral morphology) and aortic wall enhancement outside the hematoma indicates the presence of adventitial inflammation.
- MRI findings.
  - *TSE sequences*: There is hyperintensity on T2w sequences in cases of acute hematoma, with intermediate intensity if it is subacute-chronic. The T1 signal is useful in monitoring the process of hemoglobin degradation and the stabilization of dissection (acute: isointense signal; subacute-chronic: hyperintense).
  - *PC sequences and contrast-enhanced GRE sequences*: There is no flow in the middle layer (helps to differentiate the hematoma from the dissection with slow flow false lumen).

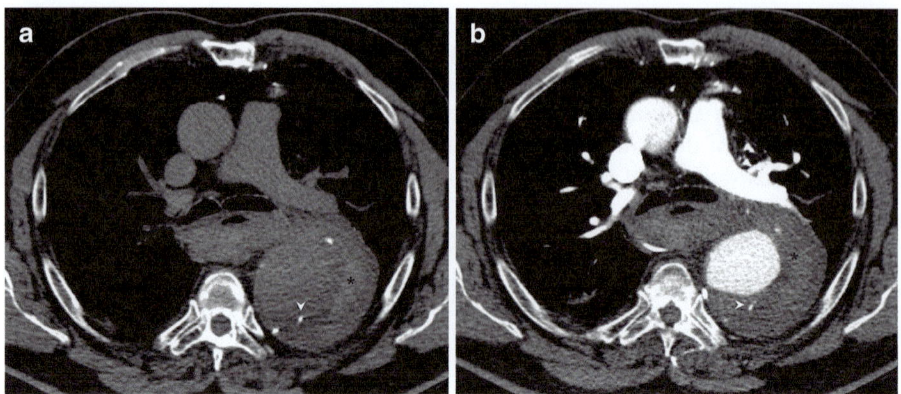

Fig. 11.14 72-year-old man with chest pain. (**a**) Pre-contrast images show a crescent-shaped area of attenuation in the aortic wall (*black asterisk*) of the descending aorta, corresponding to a hematoma in the tunica media. The intimal calcification is displaced (*white arrow head*) and abnormal circumferential thickening of the aortic wall is present. (**b**) Post-contrast images show that, unlike aortic dissection, the crescent-shaped area is not perfused by contrast and no intimal tears are seen

Differential Diagnosis

- *Aortitis*: characterized by discontinuous skip lesions (in IMH the thickening is always constant), circumferential morphology (IMH is more often eccentric); frequent involvement of other arterial branches. (Fig. 11.15).

The purpose of the report is to evaluate:

- Location of proximal and distal extremities of IMH (type A or B)
- Maximum diameter of the aorta (if ascending aorta >5 cm higher risk of mortality) and maximum and minimum size of the aortic lumen at the level of maximum hematoma thickness
- Thickness of the aortic wall (> 2 cm higher risk of mortality)
- Adventitia contrast enhancement (sign of inflammation)
- Signs of intimal ulceration (risk of evolution in penetrating ulcer)
- Supra-aortic or abdominal aortic branches extension; parenchymal perfusion

Uncomplicated IMH is treated with medical therapy and close follow-up by CTA or MRA is required according to evolution, stabilization or regression; complicated IMH is treated depending on the scenario (dissection, rupture, or aneurysm).

Penetrating Atherosclerotic Ulcer (PAU)

Penetrating atherosclerotic ulcer originates from an ulceration of an atheromatous plaque that damages the inner elastic layer of the aortic wall, stretches the middle layer, and yields hematoma formation in the media. The involvement of the tunica media can be complicated by dilatation or, rarely, by rupture.

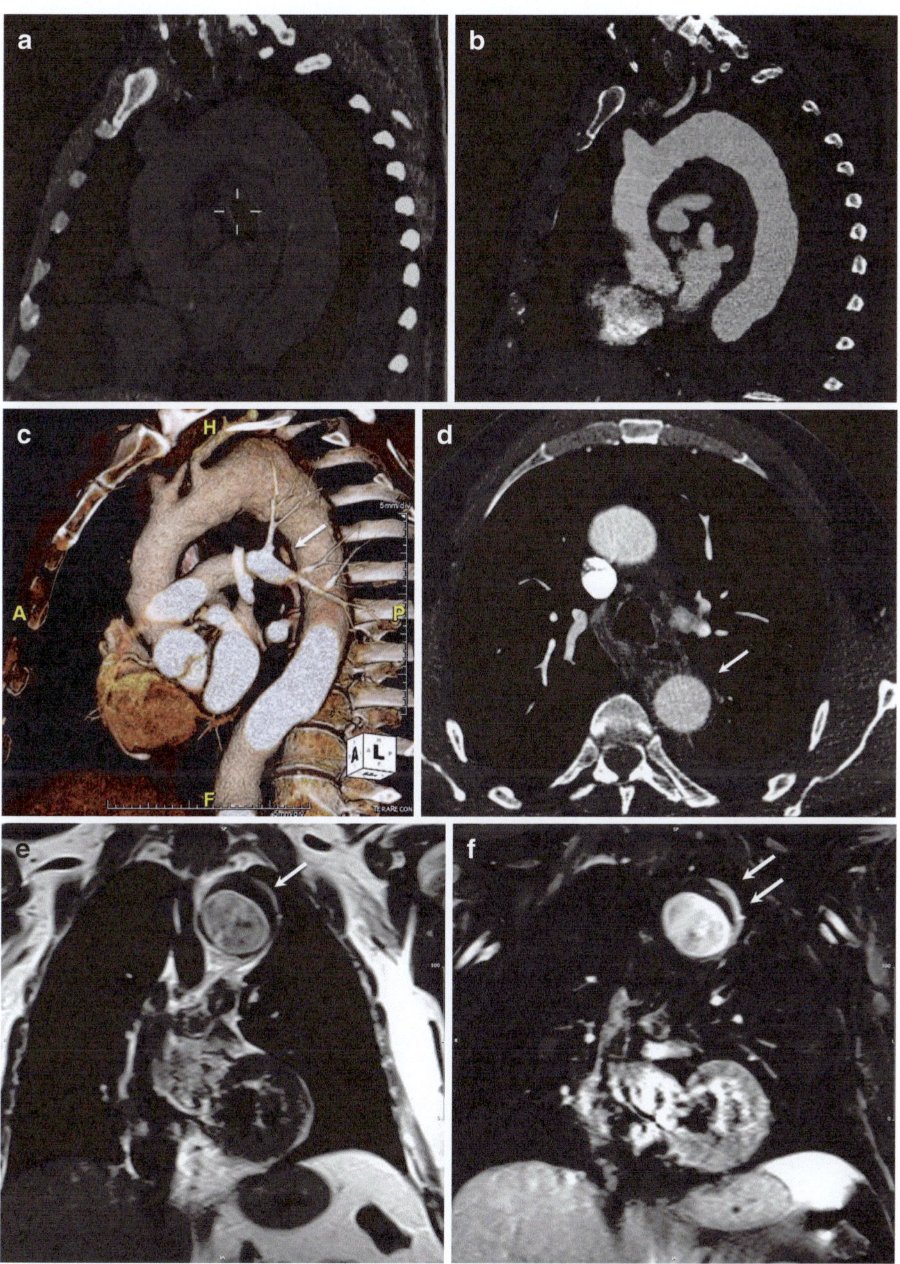

Fig. 11.15 Aortitis. (**a**, **b**): Post-contrast MPR image compared to pre-contrast image shows a thickening and hyperemia of the aortic wall. (**c**) Volume rendering reconstruction shows a small pseudoaneurysm on the anterior aortic wall, (**d**) Hyperemia of the aortic wall. MR examination confirms the thickening and hyperemia of the aortic wall on pre-contrast (**e**) and post-contrast T1-weighted sequences (**f**)

Penetrating atherosclerotic ulcers are usually seen in elderly patients with severe atherosclerosis (Fig. 11.16).

In most cases, the ulcer occurs at the aortic arch and descending thoracic aorta, while the ascending aorta is only rarely involved because the high blood flow from the left ventricle provides protection against atherosclerosis.

- On pre-contrast CT scans PAU appears as:
  - extensive atherosclerosis and IMH
  - displaced intimal calcifications
- On contrast-enhanced CT scans, PAU appears as a collection of contrast material outside the aortic lumen.

PAU is usually treated with medical therapy, as type B aortic dissection; surgery is reserved for patients who have persistent pain, aortic rupture, hemodynamic instability, distal embolization, or rapid enlargement of the aortic diameter.

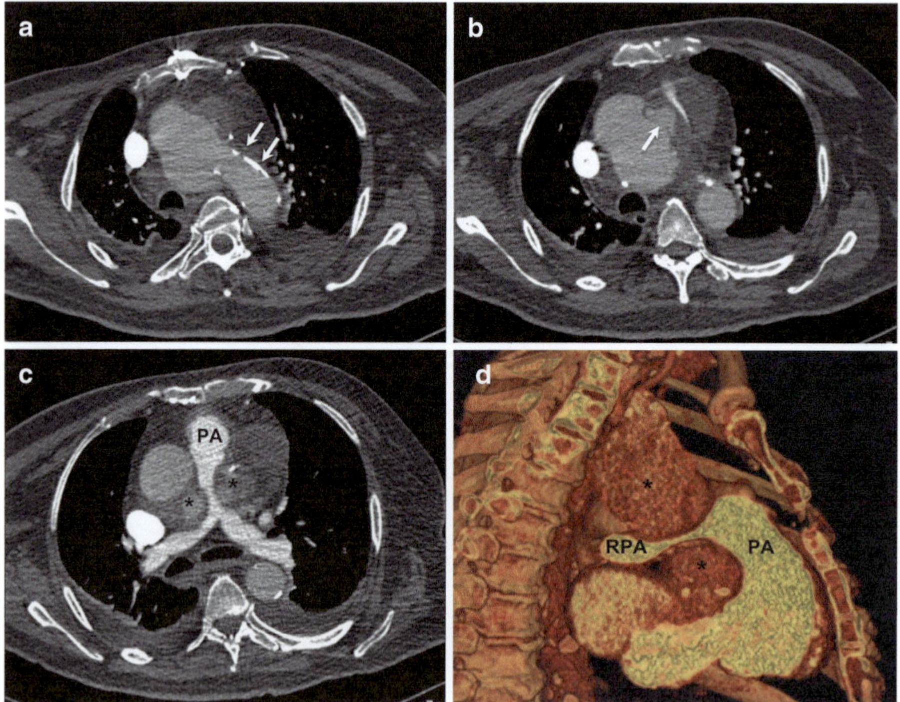

Fig. 11.16 72-year-old man with dyspnea. (**a**) Extensive atherosclerotic calcifications of the aortic arch (*arrows*), (**b**) Disruption of the aortic wall (*arrow*), (**c**) Hematoma (*black asterisks*) around the pulmonary artery (*PA*), (**d**) Volume rendering reconstruction shows the PA compressed by the hematoma

Aortic Injury from Blunt Trauma

Traumatic blunt events as road accidents, falls from heights, or explosions can be a cause of aortic damage. The aortic portions more exposed to impact forces are the ligamentum arteriosum insertion site, the aortic root, and the thoraco-abdominal passage site.

The isthmus is the most common site of aortic injury (90% of cases) that can be a pseudoaneurysm formation or an aortic transection. The mechanism of injury of the aortic isthmus is a rapid deceleration: the aortic arch is mobile compared to the proximal descending portion of the aorta and, when this is stretched anteriorly by rapid deceleration, the isthmus is stressed by opposite forces. An anteroposterior compressive force between the manubrium, first rib and medial clavicle, can push the aorta posteroinferiorly against the thoracic spine ("osseous pinch").

- Types of injuries.
  - *Pseudoaneurysm*: it is a contained rupture of the aortic wall. There is a perivascular hematic collection, arising from an eccentric interruption of the vessel wall, contained only by the adventitia or the surrounding soft tissue (periadventitial). It can stabilize or grow gradually over time and break years after injury.
  - *Aortic transection*: it is a circumferential tear of the aortic wall contained only by the adventitia (usually localized at the proximal portion of the descending aorta, close to the isthmus). It is mortal in almost all cases (99% mortality in the first 24 h).

Aortic injuries from blunt trauma are usually fatal (80–90%). Patients who survive may have different outcomes (from intramural hematoma to aortic rupture). The treatment, performed in emergency, can be surgical or endovascular.

- CT findings:
  - *Direct*: direct visualization of a pseudoaneurysm, sudden alterations of the aortic diameter or contour, intimal flaps, intraluminal thrombi, and contrast extravasation
  - *Indirect*: periaortic bleeding directly communicating with the aorta, mediastinal hematoma, hemopericardium, and hemothorax

Aneurysmal Disease

CTA is the reference diagnostic tool in the evaluation of aortic aneurysms: it shows vessel lumen and provides essential information for a correct pre-surgery planning (the extension and composition of the aneurysm sac, the relationship with close structures, the size and status of endovascular access).

An aneurysm is a focal dilatation of the aorta delimited by all three wall layers (tunica intima, tunica media, and adventitia) (Fig. 11.17). The maximum aortic

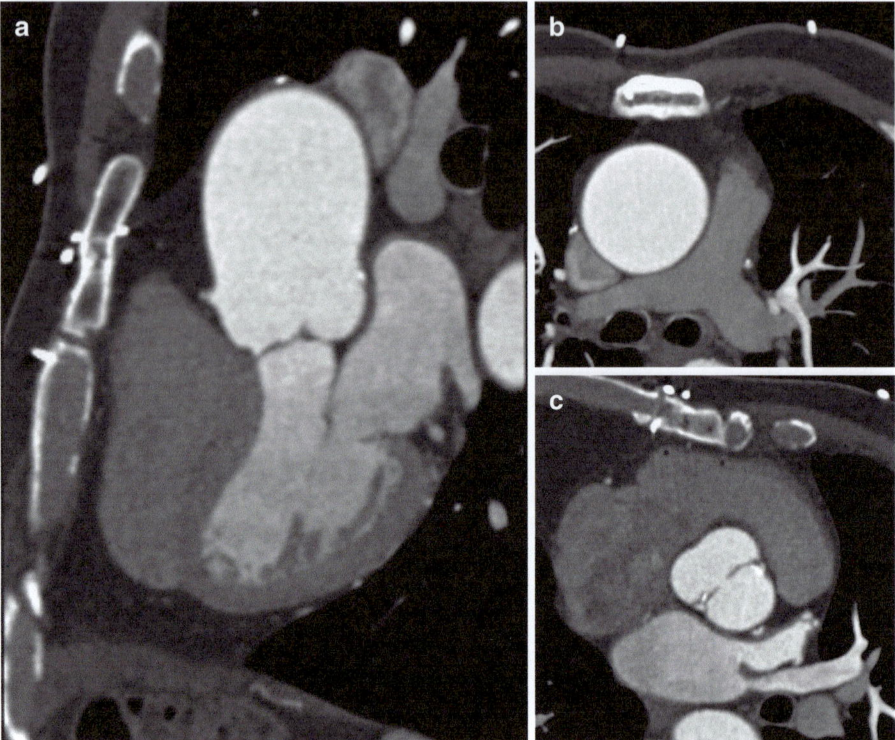

Fig. 11.17 Aneurysm of the ascending aorta and bicuspid aortic valve. (**a**) Multiplanar reconstruction (MPR) of the aortic root shows enlargement of the ascending aorta, (**b**, **c**) MPR in axial view shows the ascending aorta and the aortic valve with bicuspid morphology

diameter should not be larger than 4 cm for the ascending aorta and 3 cm for the descending portion (according to age and anthropometric data).

Atherosclerosis is the leading cause of aortic aneurysms (70% of cases) affecting more often the descending aorta. Less common causes are hereditary (cystic degeneration of the tunica media, Marfan syndrome, Ehlers-Danlos syndrome), inflammatory or infectious (syphilitic aortitis, mycotic aortitis, rheumatic fever), autoimmune (rheumatoid arthritis, systemic lupus erythematosus, scleroderma), or the presence of a congenital bicuspid valve.

Reporting an aneurysm, it is necessary to describe:

- Size, composition, and shape (saccular or fusiform).
- Measurements of residual aortic lumen if mural thrombus is present.
- Size of anchoring extremities (aneurysmal neck: aortic portion proximal and distal to the aneurysm).
- Relations with arterial branches (left subclavian artery, renal arteries, celiac trunk) and with the surrounding extravascular structures (esophagus, trachea, sternum, lung).
- Complications such as rupture or dissection. The risk of rupture increases accordingly with the size of the aneurysm (Fig. 11.18).

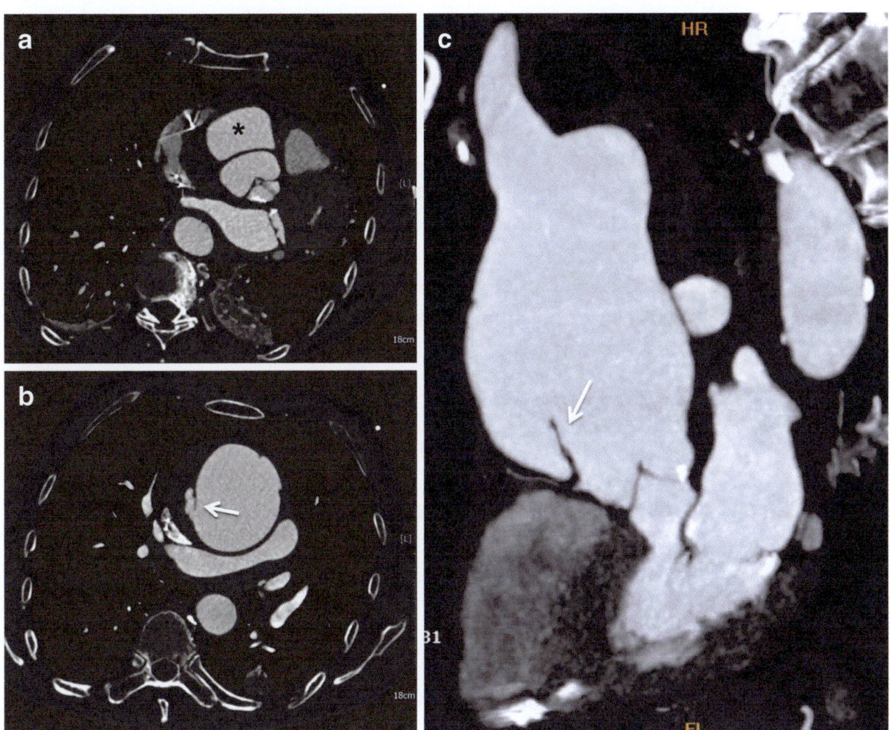

Fig. 11.18 Type A dissection in ascending aortic aneurysm. (**a**) Axial view with false (*black asterisk*) and true lumen, Axial (**b**) and MPR sagittal view (**c**) of the intimal tear (white arrow)

- CT allows to evaluate signs of:
  - *Impending rupture*, such as "sickle-shaped hyper-attenuation area" within the aortic wall or within a mural thrombus in the aneurysm (crescent sign) in pre-contrast scans (hyperdense compared to the flowing blood). It is due to hemorrhage penetrating and weakening the vessel wall, which may cause an imminent acute rupture of the aneurysm.
  - *Rupture*, such as hemomediastinum, hemothorax, hemopericardium, or esophageal fistula (pre-contrast scan is always necessary!);
  - *Contained rupture,* such as the drapery sign (loss of the fat planes between the aortic wall and the spine), periaortic hematoma, contrast medium extravasation, focal discontinuity of mural calcification.
  - *Compression of adjacent structures*: superior vena cava (superior vena cava syndrome), upper airways (dyspnea and/or laryngeal stridor), recurrent laryngeal nerve (hoarseness), or esophagus (dysphagia).

Endovascular or surgical treatment is recommended in symptomatic patients, in case of complications (rupture) or if the aneurysm is >5–6 cm (in Marfan syndrome >5 cm).

An annual CT scan is recommended for the follow-up of patients with untreated aneurysms (intervention is mandatory if it grows >1 cm per year).

Mycotic Aneurysm

All conditions (bacterial endocarditis, atherosclerosis, drug abuse, aortic trauma, systemic immunodeficiency) causing damage to the aortic wall predispose to mycotic aneurysm formation.

Moreover, the infection of the aortic wall is possible by hematogenous dissemination via the vasa vasorum or by contiguity from a nearby extravascular site of infection.

The most common responsible agents are staphylococcus aureus, streptococcus, pneumococcus, gonococcus, and salmonella.

- *CT findings:*
  It is usually of a saccular morphology, eccentric, rapidly growing, containing a thrombus and associated with wall thinning and periaortic inflammatory changes. Sometimes, they can be multiple. Rarely, it is calcified. It occurs most commonly in the ascending aorta (proximal to the region affected by endocarditis).
- *MRI findings:*
  It is hyperintense on fat-saturated T2-weighted images with enhancement of aortic wall on Gadolinium-enhanced T1-weighted images (more evident in fat suppression images).

Differential diagnosis: findings that can orient the diagnosis towards mycotic aneurysm are the fast growth (faster than atherosclerotic aneurysm), the absence of calcifications, the shape that is never fusiform, and the clinical history (fever, current or previous bacterial infection, positive blood cultures).

The treatment can be surgical or endovascular. If left untreated, it has a high mortality (67% of cases).

Pulmonary Embolism

Pulmonary embolism (PE) is the third cause of death among acute cardiovascular diseases after myocardial infarction and stroke, with an incidence of 1.5/1000 per year and a mortality rate of 10–30% if not diagnosed and treated.

It is due to the migration of solid, liquid, or air clots into one or more arterial pulmonary vessels from a peripheral site through the venous system or from the right heart. It determines a total or partial reduction of blood supply with secondary effects, such as respiratory and circulatory alterations, and may cause hemorrhagic infarction of the lung parenchyma. The most common causes of pulmonary embolism are deep vein thrombosis (DVT) and other conditions that may cause clot formation such as slow venous flow, coagulation disorders, or vessel wall injury.

Classic symptoms are dyspnea, chest pain, and hemoptysis (generally not all symptoms are present at the same time). Diagnosis is crucial for treatment and prognosis, but sometimes a clinical diagnosis is difficult because of other related factors and symptoms. Different scores such as the Wells Score enable to establish the clinical risk. Invasive measurement of the arterial pulmonary pressure using a Swan-Ganz catheter allows to classify the pulmonary embolism as minor acute, massive acute, and massive subacute. Evaluation of D-dimer levels detects the presence of a thrombotic process and has a high specificity.

Chest X-rays can identify the classic radiological findings of pulmonary embolism.

CTA is the diagnostic tool of choice in the evaluation of pulmonary embolism for its high sensitivity (64–100%) and specificity (89–100%), higher than pulmonary scintigraphy (poor reproducibility and specificity), and invasive conventional angiography. CTA shows the location and extent of clots and allows the clinician to choose the most adequate treatment; it also identifies the presence of pleuro-parenchymal lesions and signs of right ventricle overload.

MRA has a high diagnostic value in the follow-up of patients affected by PE.

In patients with contraindications to contrast media (renal failure or allergy to contrast), and with a high probability of pulmonary embolism, it may be useful to do a non-contrast scan: in such cases, clots may be seen as hyperdense.

Typical findings of acute PE are summarized in Fig. 11.19.

It is always necessary to assess if:

- PE is massive or segmental.
- Pulmonary artery is enlarged.
- The right ventricle is enlarged and if the right-to-left ventricular ratio is >0.9 in the four-chamber view.
- There is paradoxical deviation of the interventricular septum.
- There is tricuspid insufficiency with reflux of the contrast medium into the inferior vena cava.
- There are signs of DVT (in case there are, it is mandatory to include the lower limbs in the venous phase).

Acute PE usually resolves without consequences, but in 40–50% of cases CTA may detect residual clots. In patients with larger clots (0.1–0.5%), the thrombus can undergo organization and remodeling and may cause stenosis: patients are initially asymptomatic, in time they may develop severe dyspnea, pulmonary hypertension, and chronic pulmonary heart disease. CTA has a sensitivity and specificity of 95% in diagnosing chronic pulmonary embolism and is able to differentiate acute PE from chronic PE.

Risk stratification of the patients, by measuring the arterial pressure and evaluating the function of the right ventricle, enables to select the best treatment:

- In patients presenting with normal arterial pressure and right ventricular function, anticoagulant therapy is administered, and an inferior vena cava filter is placed to prevent recurrences, in case DVT is present.
- In patients affected by hypotension, the therapy is thrombolysis and embolectomy.

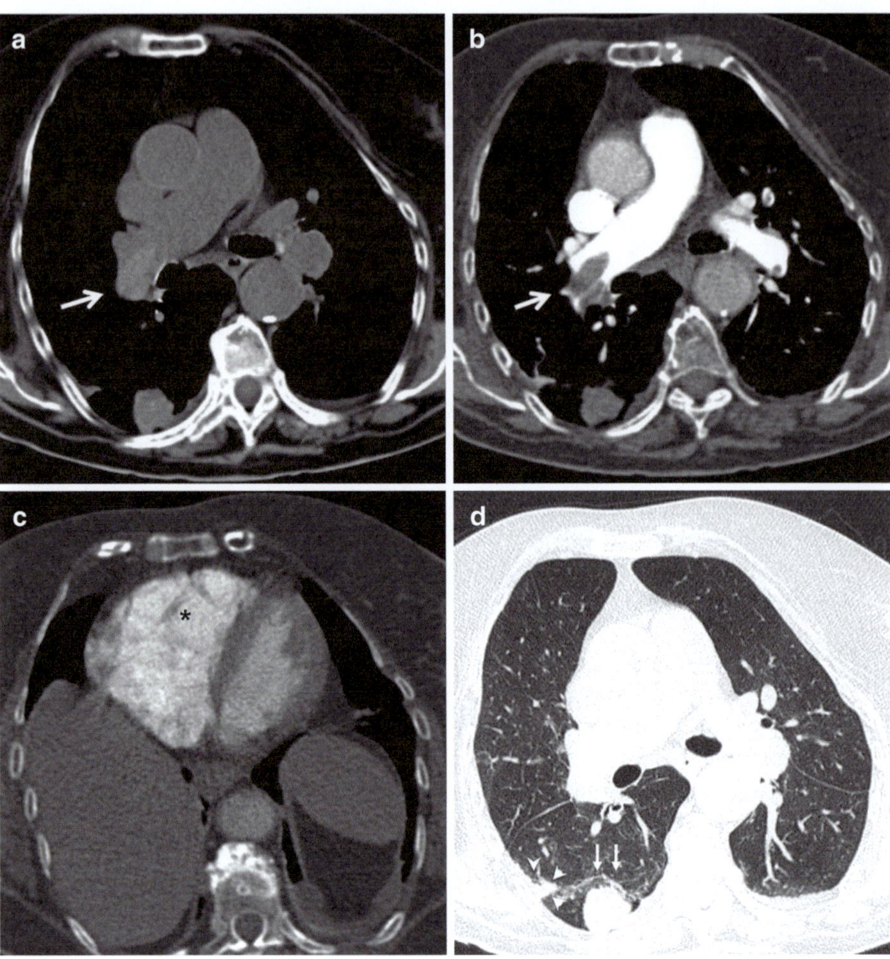

Fig. 11.19 78-year-old woman with dyspnea. (**a**) Pre-contrast scan shows a hyperdensity in the right pulmonary artery (*white arrow*), suspicious for a clot, (**b**) Contrast administration confirms the clot presence (*white arrow*); (**c**) Enlargement of right ventricle and right atrium *(black asterisk)*, (**d**) Pulmonary infarction (*white arrowheads*) and a solid mass (*white arrows*)

Pulmonary Hypertension

Pulmonary hypertension is an increase in mean arterial pressure in the pulmonary circulation greater than 25 mmHg at rest and greater than 30 mmHg after exercise, with an increased pulmonary vascular resistance. It may be idiopathic or secondary to PE, congenital diseases, infections or lung diseases, and is associated with high morbidity and mortality. Symptoms range from asthenia to dyspnea secondary to cardiac failure. Diagnosis is made evaluating hemodynamic parameters, clinical history, respiratory function tests, and radiological and histological findings.

CTA has a high positive predictive value (>95%) and specificity (>89–90%) in the evaluation of signs of pulmonary hypertension. Radiologic findings of pulmonary hypertension are summarized in Fig. 11.20.

MR evaluation of the heart includes:

- Fat-suppressed T2-weighted sequences to detect myocardial edema, if present
- T1-weighted sequences to see the morphology of the heart and great vessels
- Angiographic sequences to assess pulmonary vessels
- Post-contrast T1-weighted sequences to delineate the presence of right myocardial wall fibrosis

The goal of treatment is to treat the heart failure. Pharmacologic treatment includes positive inotropic drugs, diuretics, oxygen therapy, and anticoagulants to prevent thromboembolic events.

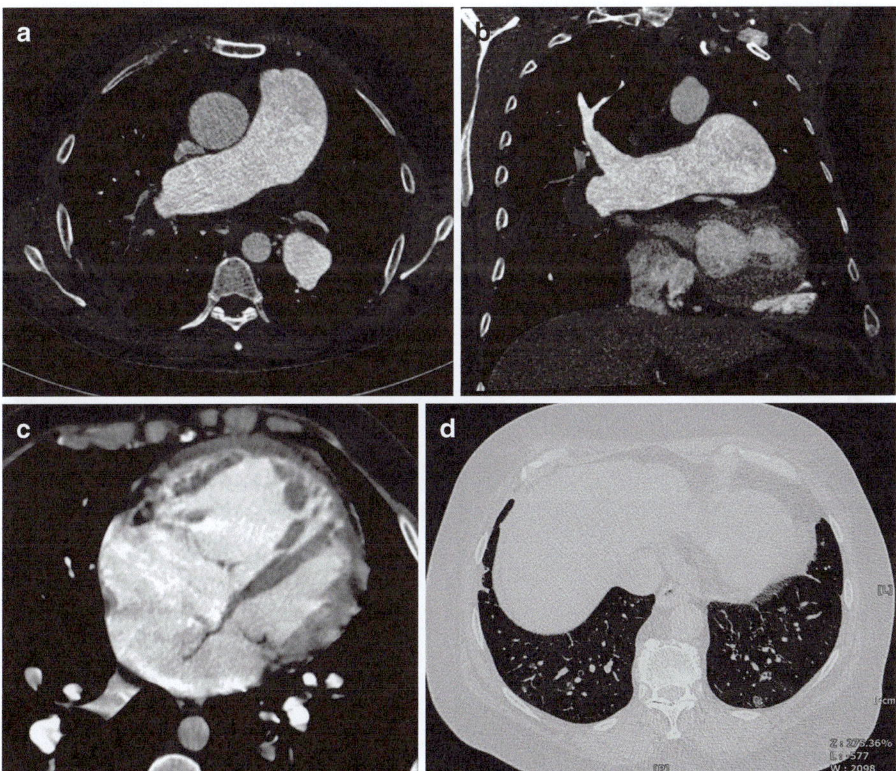

Fig. 11.20 (**a**, **b**) Enlargement of the main pulmonary trunk with intraluminal clots, associated with enlargement of the right and left pulmonary arteries and pulmonary infarction, (**c**) Enlargement of the right heart and right ventricular myocardial wall hypertrophy, (**d**) Mosaic pattern of lung attenuation

Idiopathic Pulmonary Arterial Hypertension

Idiopathic pulmonary arterial hypertension is a type of pulmonary arterial hypertension that is not easy to detect based on clinical and radiological signs. It is more frequent in young women (20–45 years), presenting with dyspnea (60% of patients), fatigue, angina, syncope, and cor pulmonale. The average delay between the onset of symptoms and diagnosis is 2 years, with a poor prognosis at 5 years (34%). The pathogenesis of idiopathic pulmonary arterial hypertension involves genetic predisposition, endothelial cell dysfunction, abnormalities in vasomotor control, thrombotic obliteration of the vascular lumen, and vascular remodeling. The most specific anatomopathological finding is plexogenic arteriopathy (detectable in 75% of cases), but it may not be easy to differentiate in situ thrombosis of peripheral vessels from chronic thromboembolic occlusion.

The most important findings of idiopathic pulmonary hypertension (Fig. 11.21) are:

- Enlargement of the main pulmonary trunk with no intraluminal clots (they may be present only in case of severe disease, associated with enlargement of the right and left pulmonary arteries)

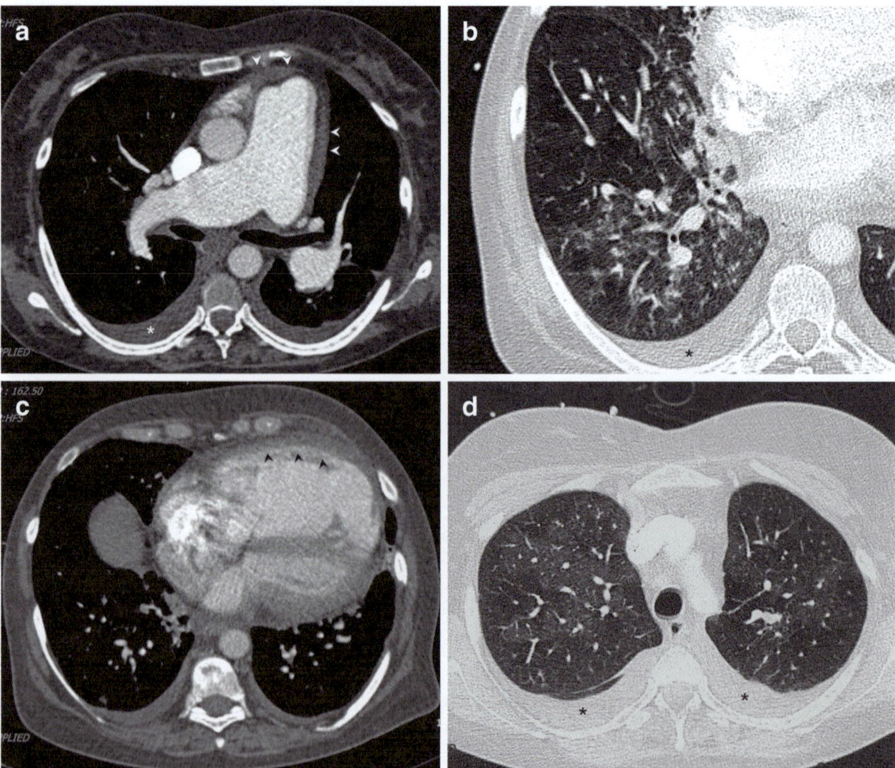

Fig. 11.21 (**a**) Enlargement of the main pulmonary trunk with no intraluminal clots and pericardial effusion (*white arrowheads*), (**b**) Small and tortuous peripheral vessels, known as plexogenic arteriopathy, (**c**) Enlargement of the right heart with myocardial hypertrophy (*black arrowheads*), (**d**) Mosaic pattern of lung attenuation

- Plexogenic arteriopathy (small and tortuous peripheral vessels)
- Segmental and subsegmental vessels presenting reduced caliber

Secondary findings are widening of the right heart, pericardial effusion, and a mosaic attenuation pattern of lung parenchyma.

When assessing the pulmonary vessels on CTA and MRA, the following must be evaluated:

- Transverse diameter of ascending aorta and pulmonary artery
- Pulmonary artery to ascending aorta ratio (P/A = 0.9)
- Transverse diameter of right and left pulmonary artery
- Presence of intraluminal clots

MRA examination allows to evaluate the morphology of the right ventricle, the left and right ventricular function, the dimensions and ratio of the right and left ventricles, the presence of pleural and pericardial effusion, and myocardial delayed enhancement (Fig. 11.22).

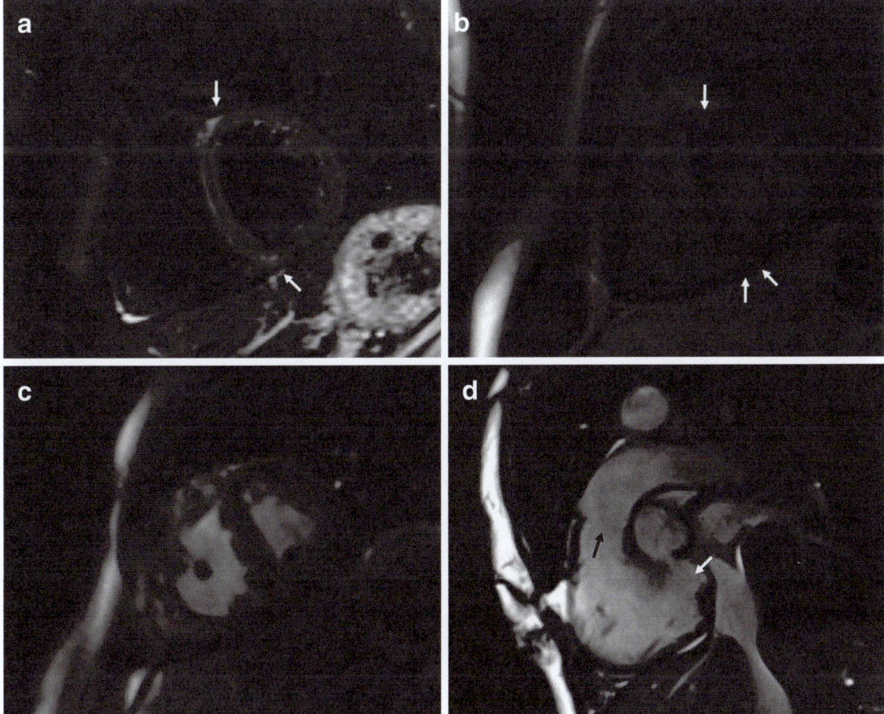

Fig. 11.22 MR sequences to assess pulmonary hypertension. (**a**) STIR (Short-Tau Inversion Recovery) sequences in the axial plane to assess the presence of myocardial edema (*arrows*), (**b**) Same plane on T1-weighted sequences acquired 15 min after contrast administration to assess late enhancement as a sign of macroscopic fibrosis (*arrows*), (**c**) Cine images to assess right and left ventricular function and flattening of the interventricular septum, (**d**) Inflow (*white arrow*) and outflow (*black arrow*) view of right ventricle

Suggested Readings

Hanneman K, Newman B, Chan F. Congenital variants and anomalies of the aortic arch. Radiographics. 2016;37(1):32–51.

Hou DJ, et al. Clinical utility of ultra high pitch dual source thoracic CT imaging of acute pulmonary embolism in the emergency department: are we one step closer towards a non-gated triple rule out? Eur J Radiol. 2013;82(10):1793–8.

McMahon MA, Squirrell CA. Multidetector CT of aortic dissection: a pictorial review. Radiographics. 2010;30(2):445–60.

Steenburg SD, et al. Acute traumatic aortic injury: imaging evaluation and management. Radiology. 2008;248(3):748–62.

Wittram C, et al. CT angiography of pulmonary embolism: diagnostic criteria and causes of misdiagnosis. Radiographics. 2004;24(5):1219–38.

Taking it to the Test: Clinical Cases 12

Cristina Marrocchio, Susan Dababou, and Hans-Peter Erasmus

Case 1

A 29-year-old Tunisian man presents with a 2-month history of low-grade fever, which he noticed especially in the evenings, cough, and weight loss. In the last 2 weeks he had recurrent hemoptysis (Fig. 12.1a–c).

What is the most likely diagnosis?

(a) Bronchogenic carcinoma
(b) Pneumatoceles
(c) Lung abscess
(d) Tuberculosis

Case 2

A chest X-ray is performed for the preoperative assessment of a patient undergoing cholecystectomy. He refers a history of past tuberculosis and wood dust exposure (Fig. 12.2a, b). A CT scan is also performed (Fig. 12.2c, d)

What is the most likely diagnosis?

(a) Atelectasis
(b) Parenchymal consolidations
(c) Pleural thickenings
(d) Honeycombing

C. Marrocchio (✉) · S. Dababou · H.-P. Erasmus
Department of Radiological, Oncological and Pathological Sciences, Sapienza University of Rome, Rome, Italy

I. Carbone, M. Anzidei (eds.), *Thoracic Radiology*,
https://doi.org/10.1007/978-3-030-35765-8_12

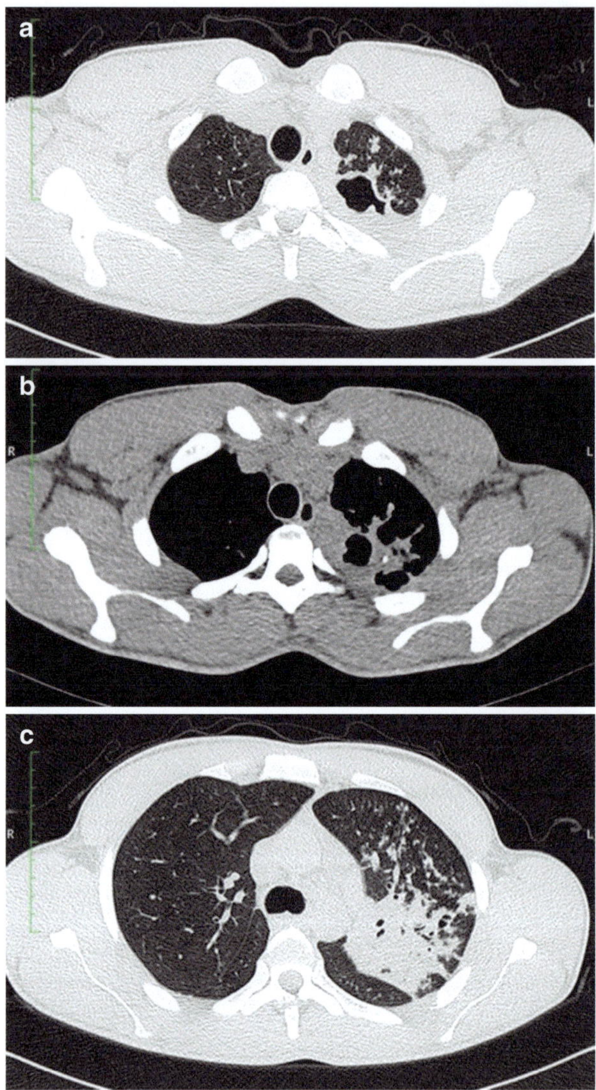

Fig. 12.1

Case 3

A 25-year-old woman presents with dyspnea and relapsing pneumothorax. Axial and coronal CT demonstrates multiple small regular cysts distributed diffusely in both lungs (Fig. 12.3a, b). Imaging of the upper abdomen shows multiple fat-containing lesions within both kidneys, most likely renal angiomyolipomas (Fig. 12.3c).

What is the most likely diagnosis?

(a) Lymphangioleiomyomatosis
(b) Cystic fibrosis

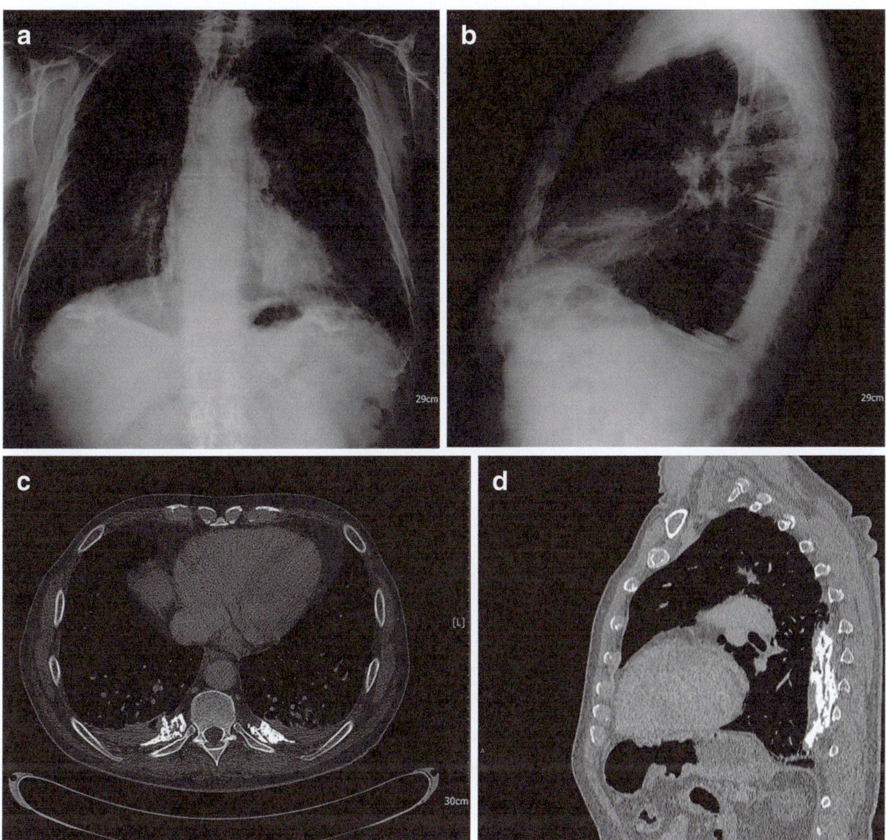

Fig. 12.2

(c) Langerhans cell histiocytosis
(d) Emphysema

Case 4

A non-smoker female patient with a recent diagnosis of Sjogren's syndrome undergoes a first CT control. She is asymptomatic (Fig. 12.4a, b).

What is the most likely diagnosis?

(a) Emphysema
(b) Lymphocytic interstitial pneumonitis
(c) Asbestosis
(d) Tuberculosis

Fig. 12.3

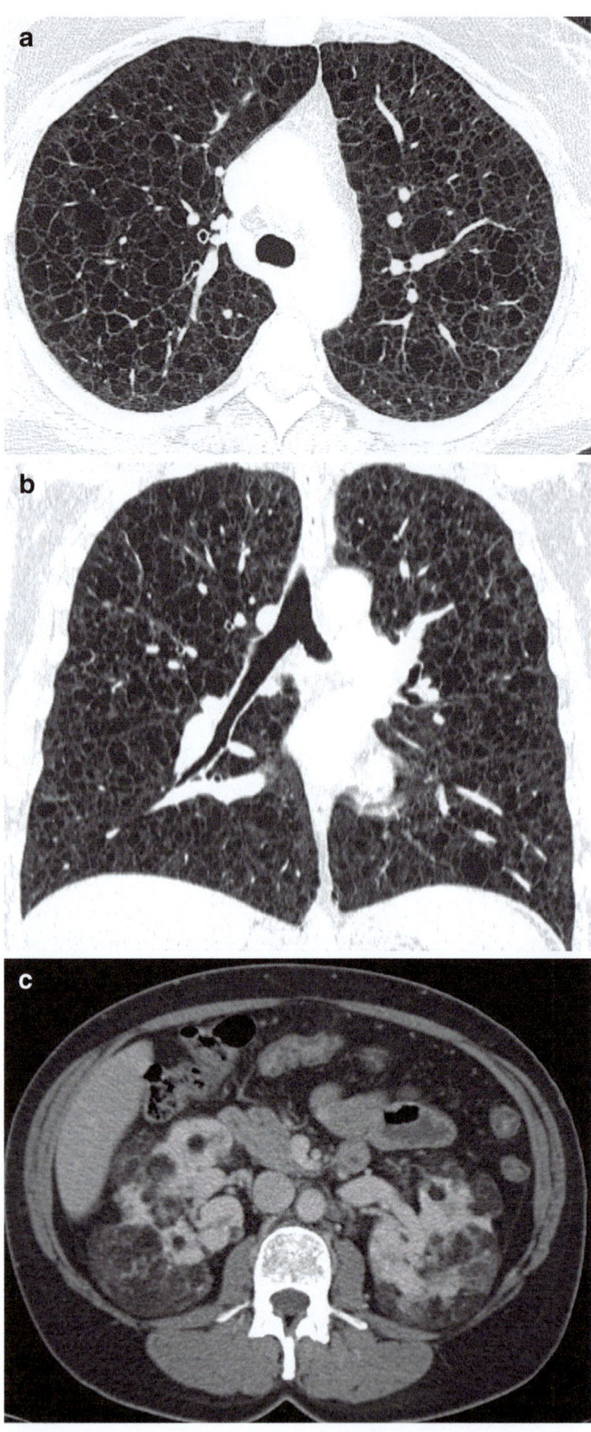

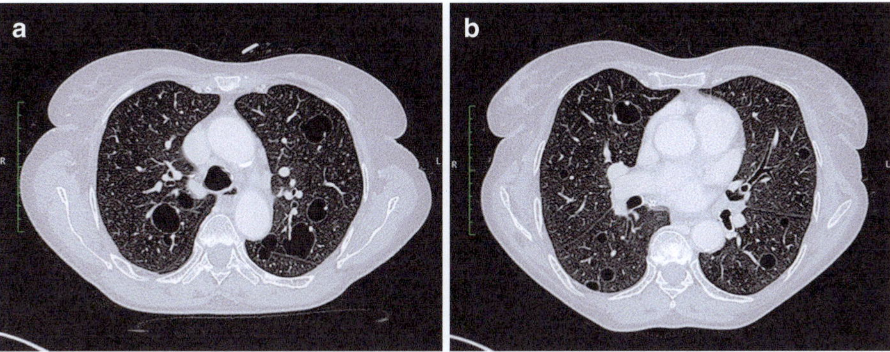

Fig. 12.4

Fig. 12.5

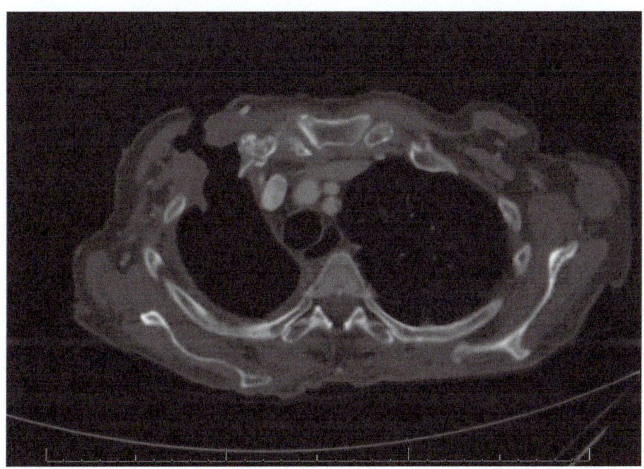

Case 5

A patient undergoes a CT scan after a right upper lobectomy for aspergilloma. What complication of the post-lobectomy space can be recognized? (Fig. 12.5)

(a) Empyema
(b) Lung collapse
(c) Pneumothorax
(d) Lung consolidation

Case 6

A 63-year-old female patient presents with a 4-month history of unwanted weight loss and cough. Her past medical history includes a papillary thyroid carcinoma treated by thyroidectomy 2 years before and radiometabolic therapy (Fig. 12.6).

Fig. 12.6

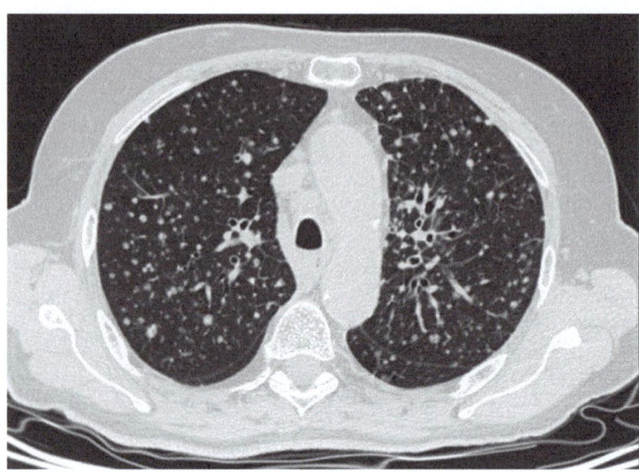

What is the most likely diagnosis?

(a) Miliary tuberculosis
(b) Histoplasmosis
(c) Sarcoidosis
(d) Miliary metastases from papillary thyroid carcinoma

Case 7

A patient presents with sepsis and acute respiratory failure after urinary tract infection (Fig. 12.7a–c).

What is the most likely diagnosis?

(a) Acute respiratory distress syndrome (ARDS)
(b) Bacterial pneumonia
(c) Heart failure
(d) Usual interstitial pneumonia

Case 8

A 60-year-old woman presents with a 1-week history of low-grade fever and persistent cough. After antibiotic therapy, the fever resolved but the cough persisted; therefore, a CT scan was performed (Fig. 12.8a–c).

What is the most likely diagnosis?

(a) Miliary metastases
(b) Miliary tuberculosis
(c) Infectious bronchiolitis
(d) Aspiration pneumonia

Fig. 12.7

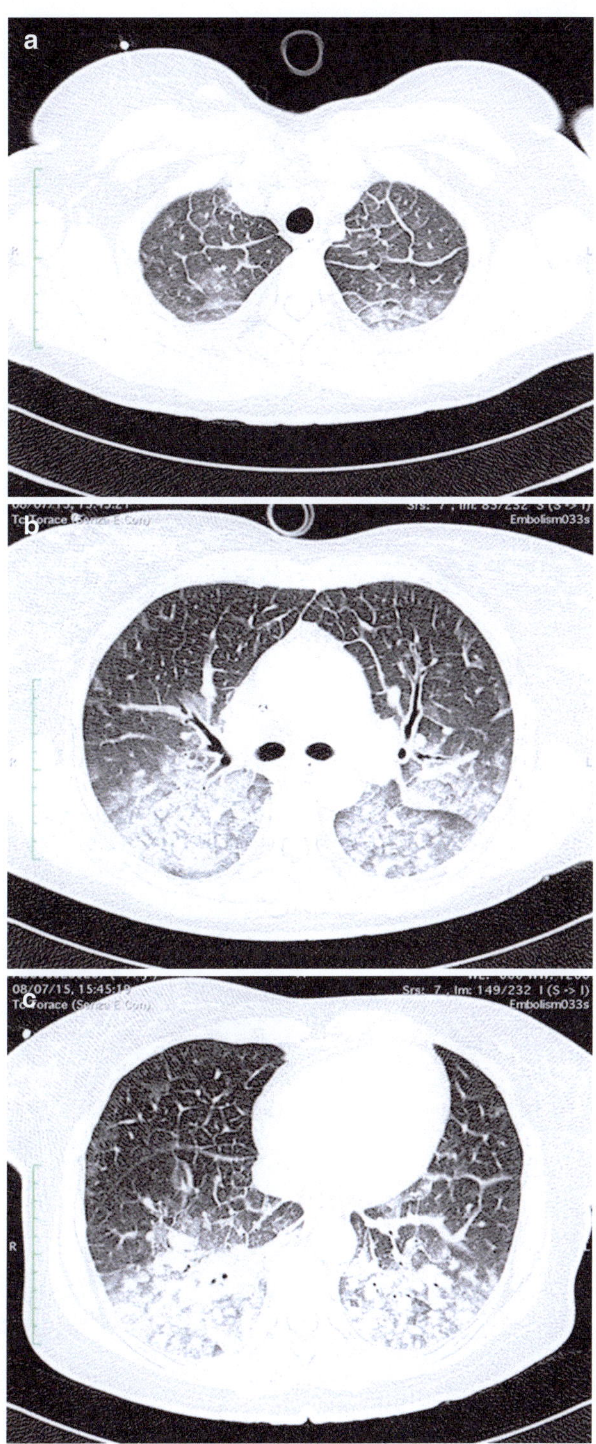
a
b
Embolism033s
c
08/07/15, 15:45:19
Srs: 7 , Im: 149/232 I (S -> I)
Embolism033s
R

Fig. 12.8

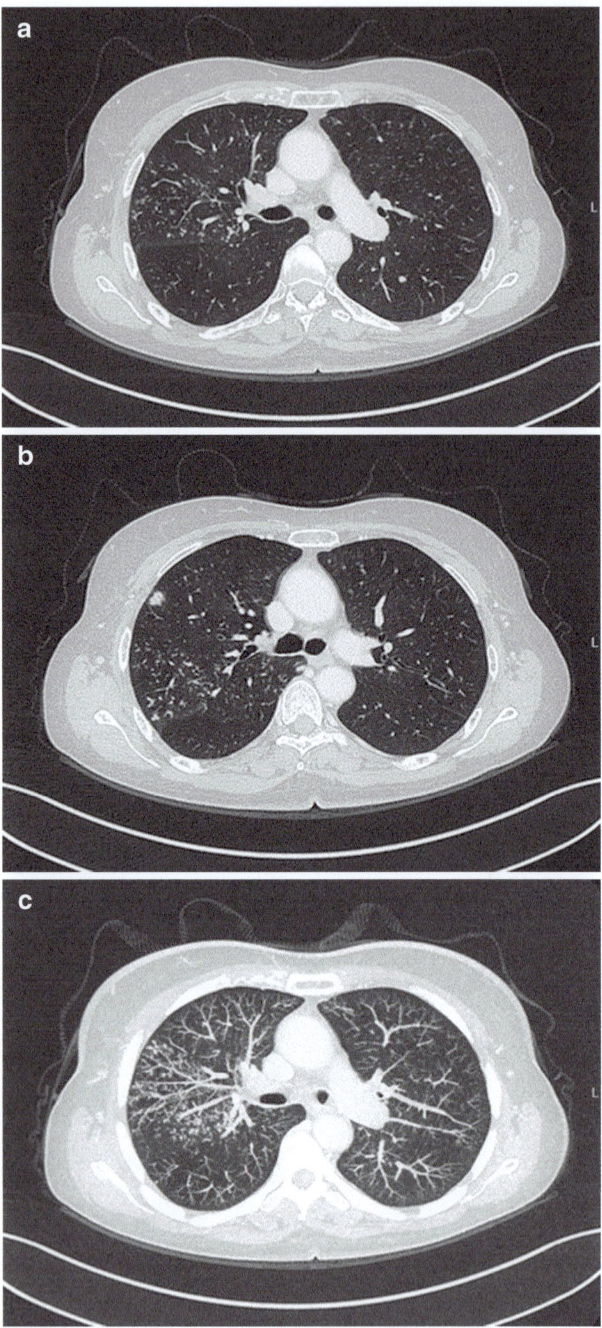

Case 9

Patient with recent-onset acute respiratory failure. On blood analysis, white blood cells are within the normal range; on white blood cell differential there is lymphopenia (about 300 total lymphocytes) (Fig. 12.9a–c).

What is the most likely diagnosis?

(a) Acute respiratory distress syndrome (ARDS)
(b) Pneumocystis pneumonia
(c) Hypersensitivity pneumonitis
(d) Pulmonary hemorrhage

Fig. 12.9

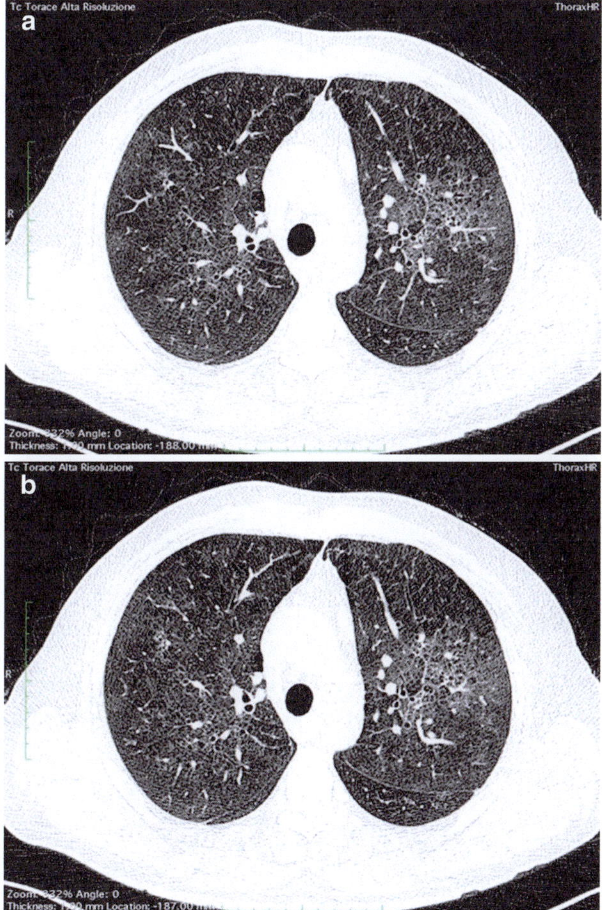

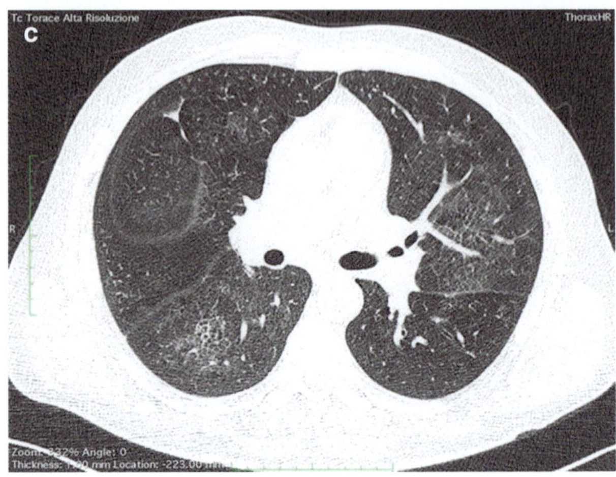

Fig. 12.9 (continued)

Case 10

A 76-year-old male patient with a past medical history of diabetes and an abdominal aortic aneurysm previously treated by endovascular repair, comes in for his routine CT follow-up. A pulmonary nodule is incidentally detected on CT (Fig. 12.10a). The radiologist decides to follow-up the nodule at 12 (Fig. 12.10b) and 24 months (Fig. 12.10c).

What is the most likely diagnosis?

(a) Bronchopneumonia
(b) Lung adenocarcinoma
(c) Parenchymal infarction
(d) Septic embolus

Case 11

A 58-year-old man presents with chest pain, worsening dyspnea and productive cough with yellowish sputum not responding to antibiotic therapy (Fig. 12.11a–d).

What is the most likely diagnosis?

(a) Pleural effusion
(b) Lung abscess
(c) Pleural mass
(d) Pleural empyema

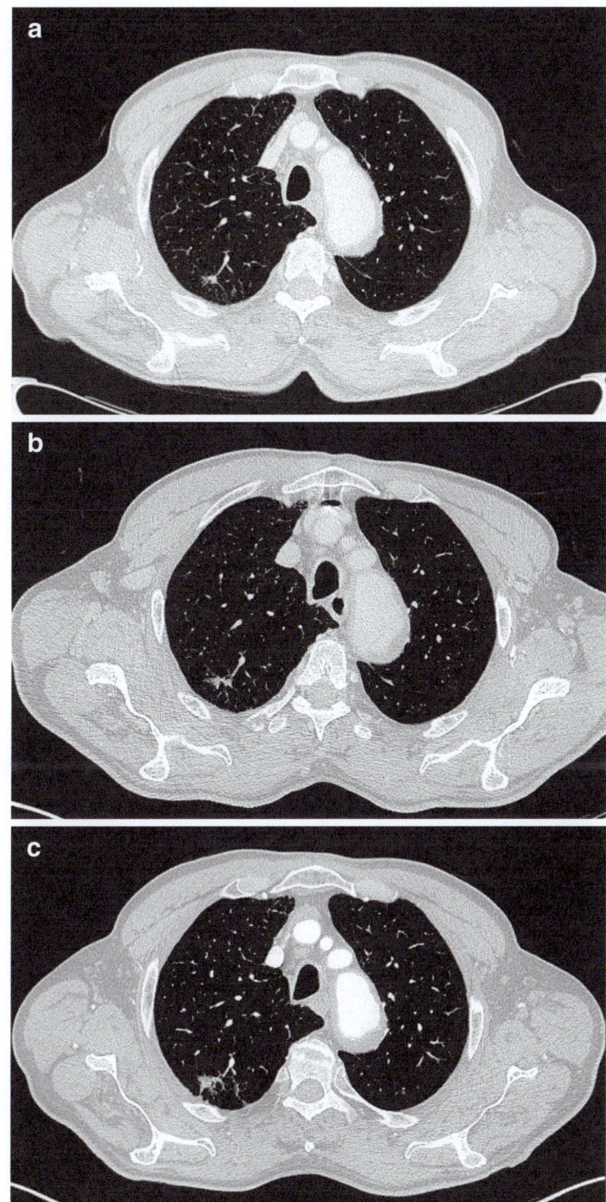

Fig. 12.10

Case 12

A patient presents with slowly progressive exertional dyspnea. On physical examination there are bilateral basal inspiratory crackles, and therefore the pneumologist asks for a high-resolution CT exam (Fig. 12.12a, b).

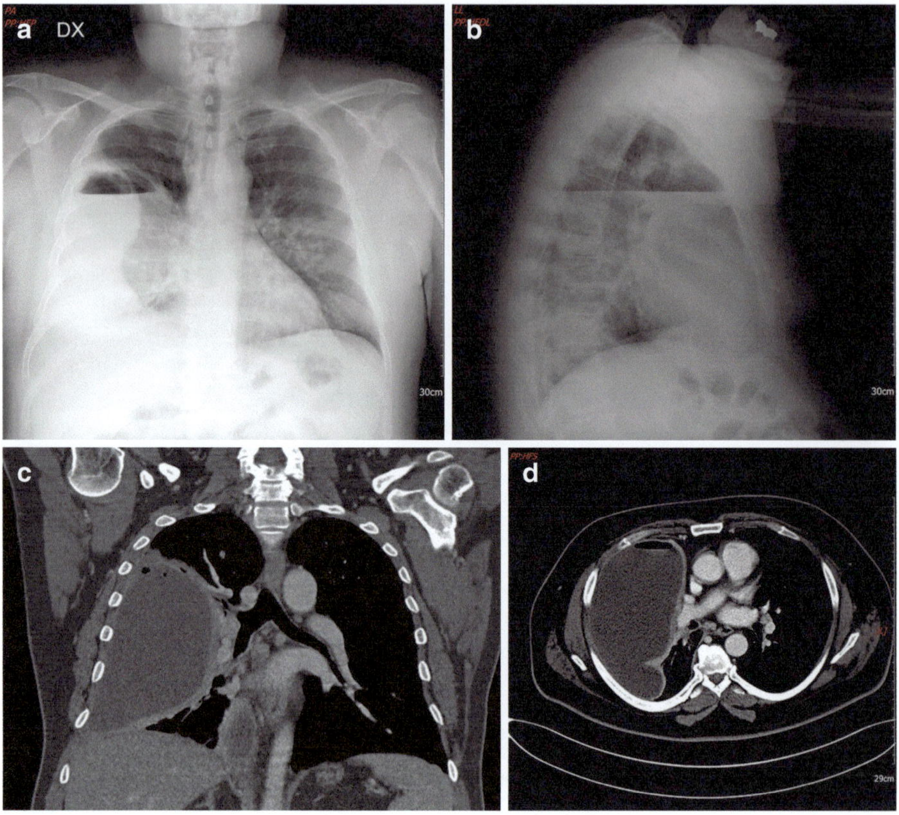

Fig. 12.11

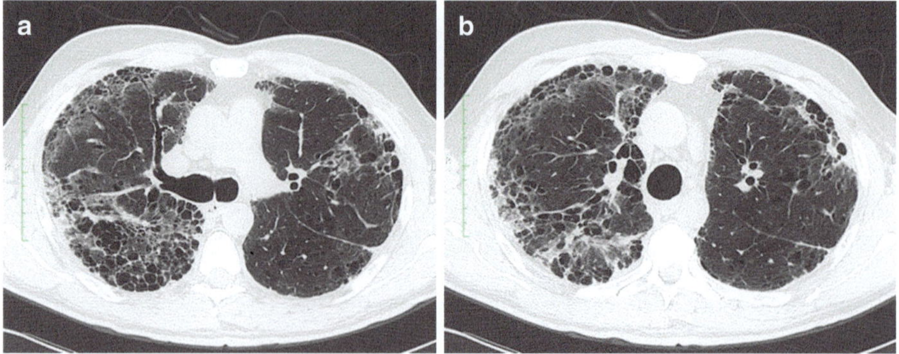

Fig. 12.12

What is the most likely diagnosis?

(a) Usual interstitial pneumonia
(b) Chronic hypersensitivity pneumonitis
(c) Cystic fibrosis
(d) Lymphangioleiomyomatosis

Case 13

A man presents with venous thrombosis of the upper limb (Fig. 12.13a–e).

In addition to subclavian vein thrombosis, what other finding is present in these CT images?

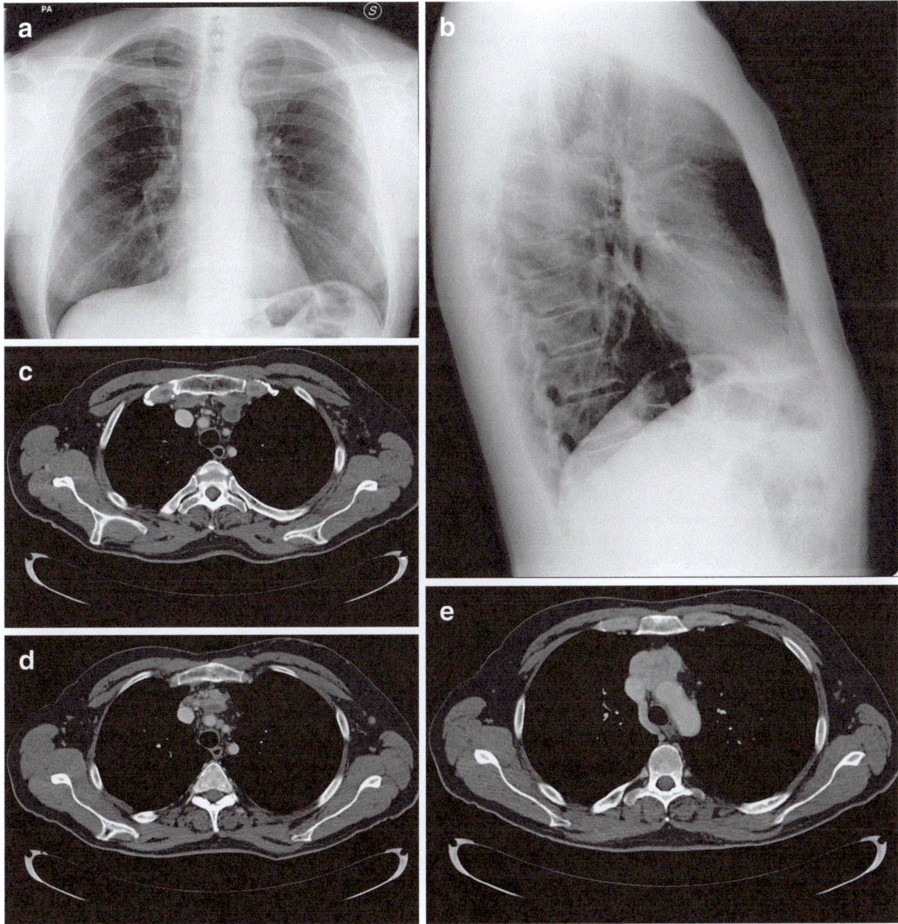

Fig. 12.13

(a) Thyroid neoplasm
(b) Aortic aneurysm
(c) Thymic carcinoma
(d) No other findings

Case 14

25-year-old smoker woman with recent onset of dyspnea and weight loss (Fig. 12.14a, b).

What is the most likely diagnosis?

(a) Langerhans cells histiocytosis
(b) Cystic fibrosis
(c) Emphysema
(d) Lymphocytic interstitial pneumonia

Case 15

An 81-year-old woman presents to the emergency department with chest pain (Fig. 12.15a, b).

What is the most likely diagnosis?

(a) Aortitis
(b) Aortic aneurysm
(c) Aortic dissection
(d) Intramural hematoma with rupture of the ascending aorta

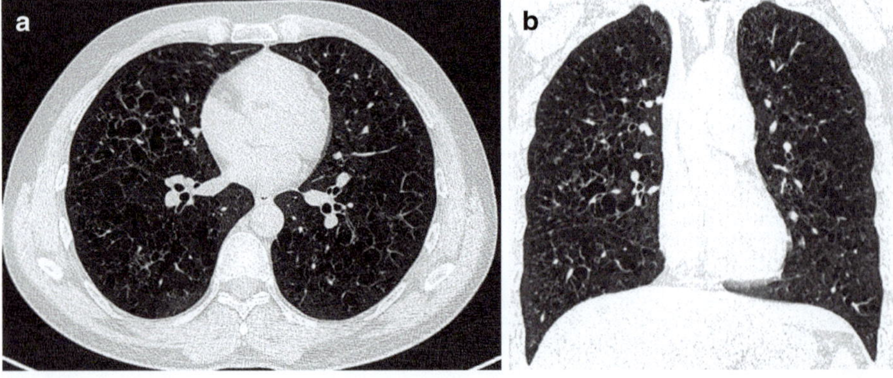

Fig. 12.14

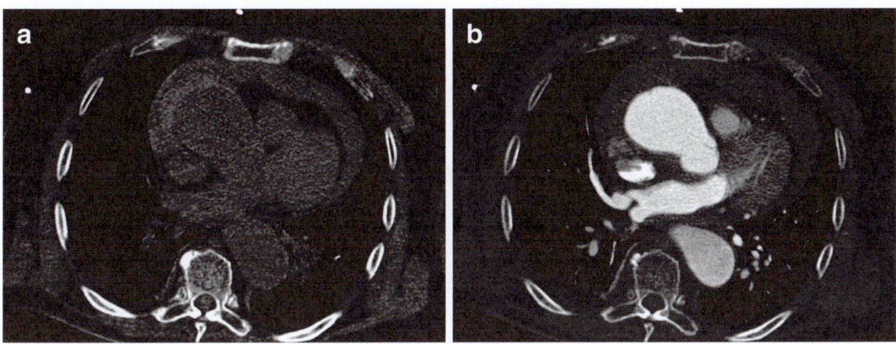

Fig. 12.15

Answers

Case 1: *d—Tuberculosis.* There is a cavitation in the apicoposterior segment of the left upper lobe with peripheral calcifications (important clue to the diagnosis of tuberculosis), surrounded by a consolidation with small peripheral tree-in-bud opacities (anterior segment of the left upper lobe, image C). In this case, the key findings for the diagnosis are: (1) ethnicity; (2) 2-month history of low-grade fever and cough; (3) apical cavitation; (4) calcification; (5) peripheral tree-in-bud, indicating bronchogenic diffusion. The patient has hemoptysis, therefore needs to be isolated.

Case 2: *c—Pleural thickenings.* The images show thickening and calcifications of the posterior part of the costovertebral pleura bilaterally. Pleural thickenings can occur secondary to chronic inflammatory diseases, usually purulent or tuberculous pleuritis, exposure to dusts (e.g., asbestos), and thoracic surgery. In most severe cases, the thickening can limit the expansion of the lungs during inspiration or cause deformities of the rib cage.

Case 3: *a—Lymphangioleiomyomatosis.* Multiple thin-walled cysts throughout the lungs, with a uniform distribution. Pneumothorax is a frequent complication. Renal angiomyolipomas are the most common abdominal findings.

Case 4: *b—Lymphocytic interstitial pneumonitis.* The images show scattered thin-walled cysts deep within the lung parenchyma, usually perivascular, with variable size within 30 mm. This finding in a patient with Sjogren's syndrome is highly suspicious for the diagnosis of lymphocytic interstitial pneumonitis. Other signs can be the presence of ground-glass opacities, centrilobular nodules, septal thickening, and thickening of bronchovascular bundles.

Case 5: *a—Empyema*, treated with open-window thoracostomy

Case 6: *d—Miliary metastases from papillary thyroid carcinoma*

Case 7: *a—Acute respiratory distress syndrome (ARDS).* Images show septal thickening, lung consolidation, and ground-glass opacities with a gravitational distribution. These signs, in the clinical settings of sepsis and in the absence of pleural effusion and heart dilatation, are consistent with diagnosis of ARDS.

Case 8: *c—Infectious bronchiolitis.* There are numerous tree-in-bud opacities in the posterior segment of the right upper lobe. They can be better appreciated in the axial MIP reconstruction in image C.

Case 9: *b—Pneumocystis pneumonia.* Thickening of intra- and interlobular septa with superimposed ground-glass opacities is called crazy paving. This sign, in the presence of lymphopenia and acute onset is highly suspicious for the diagnosis of Pneumocystis pneumonia.

Case 10: *b—Lung adenocarcinoma*

Case 11: *d—Pleural empyema.* On the right, there is a loculated pleural effusion lined by a thickened pleura and with an air-fluid level. Pleural empyema is a purulent pleural effusion, often unilateral. Symptoms can mimic a nonspecific pulmonary infection. It requires a prompt diagnosis and treatment as it is potentially lethal. The definite diagnosis requires thoracentesis and a microbiological analysis of the pleural fluid.

Case 12: *a—Usual interstitial pneumonia.* Asymmetric involvement of lung parenchyma with architectural distortion, traction bronchiectasis, and honeycombing modification, better visible on the right lower lobe.

Case 13: *c—Thymic carcinoma.* Note that the CXR is essentially negative.

Case 14: *a—Langerhans cells histiocytosis.* Axial and coronal CT images show multiple bilateral cysts with bizarre shapes, predominantly in the upper and middle lung zones, sparing the costophrenic angles.

Case 15: *d—Intramural hematoma with rupture of the ascending aorta.* Hemopericardium is consistent with a rupture of the ascending aorta into the pericardium.

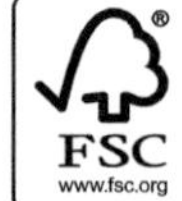

MIX
Papier aus verantwortungsvollen Quellen
Paper from responsible sources
FSC® C105338

If you have any concerns about our products,
you can contact us on
ProductSafety@springernature.com

In case Publisher is established outside the EU,
the EU authorized representative is:
Springer Nature Customer Service Center GmbH
Europaplatz 3, 69115 Heidelberg, Germany

Printed by Libri Plureos GmbH
in Hamburg, Germany